Healthcare Supply Chain

at the Intersection of Cost, Quality, and Outcomes

The Essential Guide, First Edition

Developed by GNYHA Ventures, Inc.,
and Implemented by Nexera, Inc.

Christopher J. O'Connor,
Consulting Editor

With Foreword by
Lee H. Perlman

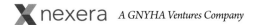

© 2015 GNYHA Ventures, Inc.
New York, NY 10019

For information on bulk purchases, please contact
gnyhapress@gnyha.org.

Printed in the United States of America
First Printing May 2015

ISBN:
978-0-9962267-4-5

Library of Congress Control Number: 2015939370

555 West 57th Street | New York, NY 10019 | nexerainc.com
Follow us on: @nexerainc /company/nexera-inc

Table of Contents

Foreword

Healthcare is a complicated set of systems and processes, but at its core, it's about the two things hospitals need to care for patients: staff and "stuff." The goal of supply chain professionals, therefore, is to ensure that their institutions have the right products at the right time for the right patient. While this mission is not new, the stakes have never been higher; health reform has ushered in a new world order of evidence-based, outcomes-driven medicine that places a premium on getting it right *at the right price*. These high stakes are creating an unprecedented opportunity for supply chain leaders to marry the business and science of healthcare to drive smarter, safer, more successful purchasing decisions.

For years, the hospital supply chain was considered transactional—its center was the office next to the loading dock, and its staff tallied inventory and completed purchase orders. The supply chain of today must be strategic, focusing on the intersection of healthcare cost, quality, and outcomes (CQO). The GNYHA Ventures family of companies has answered this call, adopting CQO[1] as its service model for hospitals and health systems around the country.

What does this model entail? *Cost*—or at least the cost of materials and equipment—has long been an area of supply chain management. CQO, however, considers all costs associated with delivering patient care and

---

[1]The Association for Healthcare Resource and Materials Management (AHRMM), a personal membership group of the American Hospital Association, launched the CQO Movement in January 2013 to encourage a more cross-disciplinary approach to healthcare supply chain management.

supporting the care environment. *Quality* refers to patient-centered care aimed at achieving the best possible clinical outcomes. *Outcomes* concern financial reimbursements driven by outstanding care at the appropriate cost. The alignment of these three factors will allow healthcare providers to deliver better care more efficiently and effectively.

Why focus on the supply chain? Quite simply, the supply chain factors into nearly every department and transaction at a hospital. Whether working with physicians and nurses on the selection of medical devices or clinical products, or managing department spending within the budgets set by hospital C-suites, supply chain executives work collaboratively across disciplines to affect—though sometimes indirectly—nearly every step of patient care delivery. From the pens used to fill out intake forms to the wheelchairs used at discharge, all hospital purchases are managed through the supply chain.

Under a CQO approach, supply chain management is elevated to a strategic level. By implementing various technologies, supply chain professionals can track patient outcomes metrics, weighing results against various clinical inputs, and monitoring effects of cost-avoidance through measures like safety needles or lower blood utilization. With these data, the supply chain can become a valuable partner in reviewing clinical protocols, product selection, and inventory management processes, identifying where hospitals can improve care and lower costs.

This book is designed to introduce the CQO model and its benefits. In addition, the team at GNYHA Ventures, led by our consultants at Nexera, Inc.[2], have created the Hospital Supply Chain Performance Self-Assessment™. This tool enables hospital and health system leaders to evaluate the performance of their supply chains against focus areas that play key roles in influencing cost, quality, and outcomes. We intend for supply chain professionals and hospital executives to use the tool to formulate supply chain performance improvement plans under a CQO approach.

---

[2]Nexera, Inc., GNYHA Ventures' supply chain management and operations efficiency company, serves as the lead sponsor of this book and administers the Hospital Supply Chain Performance Self-Assessment detailed in this text.

Supply chain professionals in today's healthcare environment have both the opportunity and responsibility to facilitate better care delivery and lower costs. We sincerely hope that this book helps you develop a CQO strategy, bring your institution's stakeholders together in a collaborative way, and enhance the strategic contributions of supply chain in the new value-based, data-driven healthcare environment.

Lee H. Perlman, FACHE
President, GNYHA Ventures, Inc.
Chief Financial Officer and Executive Vice President, GNYHA

Acknowledgments

This book and the companion online Hospital Supply Chain Performance Self-Assessment™ ("Self-Assessment") are the products of nearly two years of intensive, collaborative work by more than 40 current and former staff members of the Greater New York Hospital Association (GNYHA); GNYHA Ventures, Inc. (GNYHA's business arm); and, most importantly, two companies from the GNYHA Ventures family, namely GNYHA Services, Inc., our acute care group purchasing organization, and Nexera, Inc., our healthcare consulting firm, which has particular expertise in hospital supply chain operations. This team's deep knowledge of hospital operations in general, and hospital supply chain in particular, was instrumental in beginning to concretely define the relationship between supply chain operations and a hospital's cost, quality, and outcomes. This led to the development of tools and strategies that can be used by hospital and health system executives—administrative *and* clinical—to assess the performance of their institution's supply chain and take explicit steps to address areas of weakness with the goal of improving cost, quality, and outcomes.

Three distinct but interrelated activities occurred in connection with this project: 1) the development of the CQO focus areas and performance levels (PLD), 2) creation of the online Self-Assessment (SA), and 3) preparation of this book (B). As the architect of the CQO concept, I want to acknowledge the efforts and contributions of all those who participated in these activities, thereby helping to move CQO from concept to reality.

First and foremost, I would like to thank GNYHA President Kenneth E.

Raske, GNYHA Ventures President Lee H. Perlman, and our board members for creating the kind of environment that welcomes, encourages, and nurtures new ideas. Their unwavering commitment, forward thinking, and willingness to invest resources in projects that have the potential to bring significant value to our members and industry make the pursuit of efforts like these possible.

Second, very special thanks go to Barbara A. Green, PhD, Senior Vice President, GNYHA Ventures; Kenneth Scher, CMRP, Manager, Nexera; and Alison B. Flynn, MHA, CMRP, FACHE, Senior Vice President, GNYHA Services and Nexera. These individuals devoted countless hours leading the project team, making substantive contributions, and managing each of the three project components.

In addition, I'd like to express my sincerest thanks and appreciation to all of the following individuals. Without their expertise and individual and collective contributions, this project would not have come to fruition.

- Kristin A. Boehm, MD, FACS, Senior Advisor, Nexera (PLD, SA)
- Carole Boutilier, RN, Consultant, Nexera (SA)
- Basia A. Bubel, MS, Analyst, GNYHA Services and Nexera (SA)
- Monica Chopra, MBA, MPH, Senior Manager, Nexera (PLD)
- Michele Chotkowski, RN, MSHN, Director, GNYHA Services (PLD)
- Amy E. Cretella, Director, GNYHA Services and Nexera (PLD, SA, B)
- Sarah Czarnowski, Junior Brand Manager, GNYHA Ventures (B)
- John DePierro, Senior Advisor, GNYHA Ventures (PLD)*
- Lisa Fishelberg, MHA, Assistant Vice President, GNYHA Services (PLD)
- Jay Fligstein, Senior Vice President, GNYHA Services (PLD)
- D. Vincent Fitts Jr., MA, Vice President, Informatics and Outcomes Research, GNYHA (PLD, SA)*
- Donna Gammarato, CMRP, Vice President, GNYHA Services (PLD)
- Martin Glick, CPA, CGMA, Vice President, GNYHA Services (PLD, SA)
- Ethan Haimm, Consultant, Nexera (SA)*
- Leslie Isenegger, EMBA, MPP, Senior Vice President, GNYHA Ventures (B)
- Michael Jones, MBA, Director, Nexera (SA)

- Salil Joshi, MS, Senior Manager, Nexera (PLD, SA, B)*
- Sheryl D. Joyner, MSW, MBA, Director, Nexera (SA)
- Dieter Klipstein, Director, Graphic Design, GNYHA Ventures (B)
- Linda Nguyen, Senior Consultant, Nexera (SA)
- Robert Karcher, MA, Vice President, GNYHA Services (PLD, B)
- Theresa King, Executive Assistant, GNYHA Services and Nexera (B)
- Roberta L. Knab, Senior Vice President, Nexera (PLD, SA)*
- Patricia McCauley, RN, MSN, Manager, Nexera (PLD)
- Thomas McLoughlin, Project Manager, GNYHA Services (PLD)
- John McNamara, MBA, CPM, Director, GNYHA Services (PLD)
- Victoria Miller, FACHE, Senior Advisor, Nexera (PLD, B)*
- Sandra Monacelli McNall, MBA, RN, CNOR, Director, Nexera (SA)
- Diane Mongiello, RN, CMRP, Vice President, Nexera (PLD)*
- Mauro Pennacchia, Director, Nexera (PLD)*
- Tina Marie Pike, RN, MSN, MBA, HCA, Director, GNYHA Services (PLD)*
- Michelle Pollack, RN, Assistant Vice President, GNYHA Services (PLD)
- Gordon Roth, Senior Consultant, Nexera (PLD, SA)
- Susan Santoro, MBA, FACHE, Vice President, Nexera (PLD)*
- Perry Sham, Vice President, Nexera (PLD, SA, B)
- Ismail Sirtalan, PhD, Vice President, Economic Research, GNYHA (SA)
- Mary Twomey, RN, Director, GNYHA Services (PLD)
- Christine Tyburczy, CMRP, Manager, Nexera (PLD)*
- Ann Vayos, CMRP, Associate Vice President, GNYHA Services (PLD)
- Shawn Varughese, Analyst, GNYHA Services (PLD)*
- Bruce C. Vladek, PhD, Senior Advisor, Nexera (PLD)
- Simone Zappa, MBA, RN, Senior Manager, Nexera (PLD)*
- David Zimba, MHA, FACHE, Vice President, GNYHA Services (PLD, OSA)
- Andrew Zockoff, Senior Consultant, Nexera (PLD)*

denotes former employee at the time of publication

Next, I'd like to express my sincere gratitude to Ilene Halem Rothman and everyone at IKM who worked with our team to develop the Self-Assessment. In addition, many thanks go to NYU Langone Medical Center and Lutheran Medical Center for testing the Self-Assessment and providing valuable feedback regarding the content and functionality of this tool.

Finally, I want to thank all of my colleagues at Association for Healthcare Resource and Materials Management (AHRMM) and all of the supply chain executives who are AHRMM members for their support of CQO. Their enthusiastic embrace of this concept has transformed CQO from a mere idea to a true national movement, one that is leading to a fundamental paradigm shift in the understanding of the role that the supply chain plays and the position it occupies in hospital and health system management.

On behalf of everyone who has been involved in this project, I am pleased to share with the hospital and health system community this book, *Healthcare Supply Chain: At the Intersection of Cost, Quality, and Outcomes* and the Self-Assessment. We hope you find these to be valuable resources as you pursue the CQO journey in your hospital or health system. In the coming months and years, our understanding of supply chain management and its impact on cost, quality, and outcomes will undoubtedly continue to evolve and mature. As this occurs, we will update these resources to ensure that they always reflect the latest evidence, thinking, and knowledge.

Sincerely,

Christopher J. O'Connor, MBA, CMRP, FACHE, FAHRMM
Executive Vice President, GNYHA Ventures, Inc.
President, GNYHA Services, Inc.
President, Nexera, Inc.

"A chain is only as strong as its weakest link."
–Thomas Reid
Essays on the Intellectual Powers of a Man
1786

"The whole is greater than the sum of its parts."
–Aristotle

Introduction

The Cost, Quality, and Outcomes (CQO) Movement, launched in 2013 by the Association for Healthcare Resource and Materials Management (AHRMM), is a conceptual framework that recognizes the central role played by the supply chain in achieving hospital/health system organizational goals with respect to delivering the highest quality healthcare in the most cost-efficient manner to achieve the best possible outcomes and, as the mantra goes, "delivering the right product to the right place at the right time at the right price."[3] The CQO Movement invokes the intersection of cost, quality, and outcomes and a more holistic view of the correlation between cost (all costs associated with delivering patient care and supporting the care environment), quality (patient-centered care aimed at achieving the best possible clinical outcomes), and outcomes (financial reimbursement driven by outstanding clinical care at the appropriate costs) as opposed to viewing each independently.[4] It is premised on the following three-part construct:

- The healthcare supply chain is a complex system of interconnected components that individually and collectively influence an organization's cost, quality, and outcomes.
- Individual supply chain components can be measured on a spectrum of performance levels, and each component should strive to operate at the top performance level.

[3] AHRMM is a personal membership group of the American Hospital Association. The CQO Movement launched in 2013 under AHRMM Chair Annette Pummel, COO, ACS, and Chair-Elect Christopher J. O'Connor, President, GNYHA Services and Nexera, Inc.
[4] "Cost, Quality, Outcomes Movement," The Association for Healthcare Resource & Materials Management, accessed October 1, 2014, http://www.ahrmm.org/ahrmm/resources_and_tools/cost_quality_outcomes/what_is_cqo.jsp.

- When all supply chain components are performing at their top levels, this signifies that each component has achieved optimal efficiency and effectiveness for its individual function, and, more importantly, that the supply chain as a whole is well positioned to support the organization's overall cost, quality, and outcome goals.

The CQO Movement also defines the role, responsibilities, and expertise needed by supply chain executives to be effective and successful in today's healthcare environment. It envisions that supply chain executives "own" the intersection of cost, quality, and outcomes. This means that they are responsible for driving the process by which strategic decisions about supply spend are made with consideration given to cost, quality, and outcomes. Ideally, they utilize an evidence-based, consensus-driven approach to enable the healthcare organization to consistently deliver the right product to the right place at the right price and in the right quantities. Moreover, supply chain executives' roles place them squarely at the convergence point of the individual supply chain components; hence, they are uniquely positioned to identify and resolve conflicts, competing priorities, actions, or decisions that hinder the optimal functioning of the overall supply chain and undermine the organization's ability to ensure the best quality care at the lowest cost.

Healthcare Supply Chain: At the Intersection of Cost, Quality, and Outcomes accompanies the Hospital Supply Chain Performance Self-Assessment™ ("Self-Assessment"), a tool developed by GNYHA Ventures and implemented by Nexera to enable hospital/health system leaders to evaluate the performance of the following supply chain management components or "focus areas." The focus areas are (in alphabetical order):

I. Continuous Process Improvement (CPI)
II. Contracting
III. Data Management
IV. Distribution
V. Education and Training
VI. Internal Controls

VII.   Inventory Management

VIII. Purchasing

IX.   Receiving

X.   Reimbursement

XI.   Requisitioning

XII.   Value Analysis

Individually and collectively, the focus areas play key roles in influencing cost, quality, and outcomes, and the Self-Assessment is intended to be used by organizations as the basis for formulating a supply chain performance improvement plan (SCPIP).

Each focus area consists of one or more attributes, and each attribute is defined by specific measures that reflect successive levels of performance ranging from Level I to Level VI, where Level VI represents optimal performance. Upon completion of the Self-Assessment, individual scores are computed for each focus area along with an overall composite score. (See Appendix A, "Methods," for further details.)

This book begins by tracing how healthcare supply chain management has evolved over time and the role that third-party payment policies have had in that evolution. It then describes the performance levels and the characteristics of organizations associated with each level. Most importantly, it serves as a roadmap for organizations that are interested in improving their supply chain performance.

Inevitably, as hospitals and health systems adapt to the dynamics of an ever-evolving healthcare environment and marketplace, concomitant changes will occur in supply chain management. As this takes place, this book and the Self-Assessment will be revised and updated to reflect changing supply chain management practices and innovations, empirical evidence that emerges about effective strategies, and other relevant developments.

Who Should Take the Self-Assessment?

To gain maximum insight into the strengths and weaknesses of the supply chain and maximum benefit from the Self-Assessment, the Self-Assessment should be taken by all hospital/health system leaders who have direct or indirect responsibility for the supply chain and/or an effect on its operations. This includes the chief executive officer/president, chief financial officer, chief operating officer, supply chain executive (often formerly known as the materials manager, purchasing director, or vice president, supply chain), chief medical officer, chief nursing officer, and chief information officer, along with the leaders of performance improvement, key clinical departments, and key support services (e.g., distribution, receiving, inventory management, central sterile processing, data management, value analysis, and education and training), given the important roles they play either in supply chain operations, as supply chain end users, or both. Using a team approach to the Self-Assessment will do the following:

- Give valuable insight into the effectiveness of supply chain operations based on input from all key stakeholders.
- Foster a better understanding by all organizational leaders of how the supply chain is connected to and integrated with the organization's total business operation–that is, all clinical and administrative units.
- Establish a basis for achieving consensus on priorities for improvement.
- Perhaps most importantly, provide the impetus for a dialogue among all key hospital/health system leaders about the fundamental and integral role the supply chain plays in achieving an organization's goals with respect to cost, quality, and outcomes.

Clearly, the value of the Self-Assessment is a function of the extent to which respondents are candid in their answers. To encourage this, all scores are reported in the aggregate to ensure the anonymity of individual respondents. Scores produced by the Self-Assessment should not be mistaken for supply chain executives' "grades." They should be regarded as a compass for identifying performance improvement opportunities that span the hospital/health system.

Scheduling the Self-Assessment

Self-Assessments are scheduled by the performance improvement team at Nexera. Once scheduled, respondents receive a link to the Self-Assessment and have up to 30 days to complete it. Each time a hospital/health system is interested in repeating the assessment, a new assessment is scheduled so that results can be reported for individual time periods and compared over time. Repeating the assessment at periodic intervals (e.g., every six months or annually) enables a hospital/health system to track changes and obtain feedback about supply chain operations to inform future performance improvement efforts.

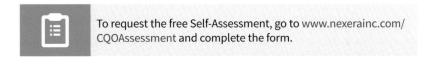

To request the free Self-Assessment, go to www.nexerainc.com/CQOAssessment and complete the form.

How Frequently Should the Self-Assessment Be Taken?

There's no limit to the number of times the Self-Assessment can be taken. It's recommended that it be taken to establish a baseline and then repeated at periodic intervals (e.g., six months or annually) to track progress.

The Self-Assessment Results Are In … Now What?

The Self-Assessment produces a wealth of information that can serve as the basis for the organization's SCPIP development. The SCPIP should be viewed as an organic document that is continually revised and updated as progress is achieved. While each SCPIP will be unique, suggested core elements include:

- The strengths and weaknesses of the current state of the supply chain. This may be based, in part, on the scores generated by the Self-Assessment for each of the supply chain focus areas.
- Priority areas for improvement. These priorities should reflect consensus among the supply chain leadership team and be tied to the organization's broader goals with respect to cost, quality, and outcomes. The priorities will be updated and reordered as projects are completed.
- A detailed work plan that spells out the steps to be taken to improve each priority area, a timetable for the requisite steps, a list of those accountable for implementation, and a list of those whose participation is needed for successful implementation.

- What resources are needed to implement the SCPIP elements.
- Expected results and how progress will be measured.

Once the SCPIP is completed, implementation begins. For most hospitals/ health systems, implementation is a complex process involving multiple departments and stakeholders. As such, it is recommended that standard project management strategies[5] be used. These time-tested strategies are particularly helpful for ensuring that initiatives stay on schedule, monitoring progress, keeping participants and others informed of project status, making course corrections on existing initiatives, and adding new projects as others are completed and/or resources permit.

Moving Up the Performance-Level Ladder

From the perspective of both the individual focus areas and the overall supply chain, the goal is to achieve Level VI performance. As a practical matter, achieving such a score is difficult given the organizational complexities typically associated with hospitals/health systems, such as competing interests, conflicting priorities, ever-changing externalities (e.g., third-party payer policies and reimbursement), resource constraints, and so forth. Nevertheless, most organizations stand to benefit significantly by taking steps to improve their performance both within focus areas and overall, as such efforts should result in incremental, quantifiable improvements. Because each hospital/health system is unique, the starting point for each organization will be a function of a host of factors. Generally speaking, however, it is recommended that most organizations address (as early as possible) three key areas—data collection/management, continuous process improvement, and value analysis. From a CQO perspective, these focus areas are important underpinnings for significant improvement and thus should be a top priority for organizations' administrative and clinical leaders.

The following sections of this book describe the characteristics of organizations at each performance level. After establishing baseline Self-Assessment scores, the supply chain executive and others responsible for SCPIP implementation can use this information to move their organization to higher levels of performance.

---

[5] See, for example, *A Guide to the Project Management Body of Knowledge* (PMBOK® Guide), 5th ed. (Project Management Institute, 2013).

Evolution of Healthcare Supply Chain Management

A look back at the approach to supply chain management in healthcare organizations finds, not surprisingly, that the strategy of hospital/health system supplies management at any given point in time has been driven largely by prevailing reimbursement policies (see Attachment 1, "Major Milestones in Healthcare Reimbursement Policies"). This section traces this evolution from when reimbursement was essentially open-ended to when cost containment became an overriding concern to today's focus on cost, quality, and outcomes.

The Origins of Health Insurance in the United States:

An Employer-Based, Cost-Based System

Between the late 1920s and the early 1970s, the basic structure of the US health insurance system was formed. In 1929, teachers in Dallas established the first insurance plan for hospital coverage,[6] leading to the creation of the Blue Cross and Blue Shield plans, which provided the earliest forms of private health coverage for hospital and physician services, respectively.[7] Tax incentives provided by the federal government in the 1940s gave rise to widespread employer-based health insurance.[8] In 1965, the federal government enacted the Medicare and Medicaid

---

[6]T. C. Buchmueller and A. C. Monheit, "Employer-Sponsored Health Insurance and the Promise of Health Insurance Reform" (NBER Working Paper Number 14839, National Bureau of Economic Research, Cambridge, MA, April 2009).

[7]M. A. Green and J. C. Rowell, *Understanding Health Insurance: A Guide to Billing and Reimbursement*, 10th ed. (Clifton Park, NY: Delmar Cengage Learning, 2010) Table 2-A (excerpts).

[8]*Medicare Hospital Prospective Payment System: How DRG Rates Are Calculated and Updated* (Office of the Inspector General, Office of Evaluations, Region IX, OEI-09-00-00200, August 2001). https://oig.hhs.gov/oei/reports/oei-09-00-00200.pdf.

programs, providing healthcare coverage to elderly and low-income Americans. During this time, hospital services were paid for by both private and public insurance programs on the basis of a retrospective, cost-based reimbursement system under which they were reimbursed for their actual costs of goods and services plus an overhead amount.[9] In this environment, there were no incentives for hospitals or other providers to manage costs, so, from a supply chain perspective, the cost and/or price of products and supplies were of little concern. Hospital storerooms were typically decentralized with multiple purchasers and supply clerks who reported to individual nursing units. Widely used items were purchased from different suppliers at different prices. It was not unusual for functionally equivalent gauze, tape, catheters, and suture items to be purchased by different departments at different prices and stored in quantities limited only by space constraints within the consuming department.[10] Supply chain management was primarily concerned with transactional metrics such as fill rates, accuracy of product orders, and timeliness of shipments.[11]

The Era of Cost Containment

This virtually open-ended reimbursement system—coupled with major advances in medical technology—resulted in rapidly escalating healthcare costs. Between 1967 and 1983, for example, Medicare's annual hospital costs rose from $3 billion to $37 billion.[12] This sparked concerns among policymakers, who began taking steps to curb growth in health spending. Their efforts embraced such payment and care delivery models as capitation and managed care, leading to the eventual adoption of the prospective payment system by Medicare, which pays hospitals flat rates based on diagnosis-related groups (DRGs).[13] In this environment, hospital purchases and procurement practices became a major focal point for hospital/health system executives, resulting in purchasing decisions that were driven largely by the cost of products and services.

---

[9] *Medicare Hospital Prospective Payment System*, 7.
[10] R. J. Karcher (Vice President, Contracting Services, GNYHA Services, Inc.), in discussion with the author, March 10, 2014.
[11] M. Darling and S. Wise, "Not Your Father's Supply Chain," Materials Management in Health Care 19, no. 4 (2010): 4.
[12] *Medicare Hospital Prospective Payment System*, 7.
[13] Prospective payment systems have also been developed for skilled nursing facilities, home health agencies, hospital-based outpatient services, inpatient rehabilitation facilities, and inpatient psychiatric facilities.

Linking Cost with Quality and Outcomes

Cost containment remained an overarching concern among health policymakers for roughly two decades. Beginning in the early 2000s, however, attention shifted to quality and outcomes in response to studies pointing to wide, not easily explained variations in quality and outcomes by procedure, provider, and geography.[14] This led to such initiatives as value-based purchasing and pay-for-performance, described as follows by the Rand Corporation:

> *Value-based purchasing (VBP) refers to a broad set of performance-based strategies that link financial incentives to providers' performance on a set of defined measures. Both public and private payers are using VBP strategies in an effort to drive improvements in quality and to slow the growth in health care spending. Nearly ten years ago, the Department of Health and Human Services (HHS) and the Centers for Medicare and Medicaid Services (CMS) began testing VBP models with their hospital pay-for-performance (P4P) demonstrations, known as the Premier Hospital Quality Incentive Demonstration (HQID) and the Physician Group Practice (PGP) Demonstration, which provided financial incentives to physician groups that performed well on quality and cost metrics. The use of financial incentives as a strategy to drive improvements in care dates back even further among private payers and Medicaid programs, with limited experimentation occurring in the early 1990s; more widespread use of P4P began to pick up steam in the late 1990s and early 2000s.[15]*

---

[14]This is an extensive literature, but see, for example, A. Donabedian, "Evaluating the Quality of Medical Care," *Milbank Memorial Fund Quarterly* VLIV, no. 3 (1966): 166–206; R. H. Brook et al., *Quality of Medical Care Assessment Using Outcome Measures: An Overview of the Method* (Santa Monica, CA: Rand Corporation, 1976) http://www.rand.org/pubs/reports/R2021z1; M. J. Pauly, "What Is Unnecessary Surgery?" *Milbank Memorial Fund Quarterly/Health and Society* 57 (1979): 95–117; N. P. Roos and L. L. Roos, Jr., "High and Low Surgical Rates: Risk Factors for Area Residents," *American Journal of Public Health* 71 (1981): 591–600; J. Wennberg and A. Gittelsohn, "Variations in Medical Care Among Small Areas," *Scientific American* 246 (1982): 120–133; J. E. Wennberg, "Hospital Use and Mortality Among Medicare Beneficiaries in Boston and New Haven," *New England Journal of Medicine* 321 (1989): 1168–1173; A. R. Tarlov et al., "The Medical Outcomes Study: An Application of Methods for Monitoring the Results of Medical Care," *JAMA* 262, no. 7 (1989): 925–930; C. M. Clancy and J. M. Eisenberg, "Outcomes Research: Measuring the End Results of Health Care," *Science* 282, no. 5387 (1998): 245–246; L. L. Leape et al., "Does Inappropriate Use Explain Small-Area Variations in the Use of Health Services?" *JAMA* 263, no. 5 (1990): 669–672; Institute of Medicine, *Crossing the Quality Chasm: A New Health System for the 21st Century* (Washington, DC: National Academies Press, 2001); and D. S. Lee et al., "Comparison of Coding of Health Failure and Comorbidities in Administrative and Clinical Data for Use in Outcomes Research," *Medical Care* 43, no. 2 (2005): 182–188.

[15] C. L. Damberg et al., *Measuring Success in Health Care Value-Based Purchasing Programs: Findings from an Environmental Scan, Literature Review, and Expert Panel Discussions* (Santa Monica, CA: Rand Corporation, Executive Summary, 2014), http://www.rand.org/pubs/research_reports/RR306.

While these initiatives had varying degrees of success, they triggered a major structural shift in the healthcare delivery system from one that was heavily reliant on hospitals and inpatient services to one that emphasized fewer hospitals, shorter hospital stays, and more outpatient and community-based care. As a consequence, the number of nonfederal community hospitals declined from 6,774 to 5,516[16] between 1975 and 2011; discharges dropped from 1,744.5 per 10,000 population in 1980 to 1,125.1 per 10,000 population in 2010;[17] hospital occupancy rates fell from 76.7% in 1975 to 66.5% in 2011;[18] average length of stay declined from 11.4 days in 1975 to 6.2 days in 2009;[19] hospital outpatient visits rose from 254.8 million in 1975 to 754.4 million in 2011;[20] the number of community health centers grew from two federally funded neighborhood health centers in 1965 to nearly 1,200 by 2012;[21] the number of ambulatory surgery centers grew from 42 in 1975 to 5,260 by 2013;[22] and the number of physician group practices (including single-specialty, multi-specialty, and family/general group practices) increased from almost 6,400 in 1969 to nearly 19,700 by 1996.[23]

Enter the Patient Protection and Affordable Care Act (ACA), the Obama administration's comprehensive health reform initiative enacted in 2010. This sweeping health reform package contained two primary goals: making health insurance coverage available to virtually all uninsured/underinsured Americans and improving the efficiency and quality of the healthcare delivery system. To accomplish these goals, the ACA does the following:

---

[16] National Center for Health Statistics. *Health, United States, 2013* (Hyattsville, MD: U.S. Department of Health and Human Services, 2014), 321, Table 107.

[17] National Center for Health Statistics. *Health*, 298, Table 95.

[18] National Center for Health Statistics. *Health*, 321, Table 107.

[19] National Center for Health Statistics. *Health*, 348, Table 108.

[20] National Center for Health Statistics. *Health*, 314, Table 100.

[21] "Press Kit," National Association of Community Health Centers, accessed March 12, 2014, http://www.nachc.com/press-kit.cfm; and *United States Health Center Fact Sheet, 2012* (National Association of Community Health Centers), http://www.nachc.com/client/documents/research/maps/US14.pdf.

[22] "History," ASPCA Ambulatory Surgery Center Association, http://www.ascaconnect.org/ASCA/AboutUs/WhatisanASC/History/; and R. Fields, "Number of Ambulatory Surgery Centers Approaches Number of Hospitals Nationwide," *Becker's ASC Review*, January 30, 2013, http://www.beckersasc.com/asc-transactions-and-valuation-issues/number-of-ambulatory-surgery-centers-approaches-number-of-hospitals-nationwide.html.

[23] Paul J. Feldstein, "Chapter 11, The Physician Services Market," in *Health Care Economics*, 7th ed. (Clifton Park, NY: Delmar Cengage Learning, 2012), 257, Table 11-2.

- Establishes a system of federal and state health insurance exchanges through which consumers can purchase health insurance.
- Promotes new models of care through such arrangements as accountable care organizations, patient-centered medical homes, and bundled and global payments.
- Fosters improved quality through pay for performance, shared savings, and hospital/physician gain-sharing programs.
- Imposes penalties for unnecessary readmissions and healthcare-acquired conditions.[24]

The implications of the ACA are far-reaching from the standpoint of both the department/division/unit responsible for supply chain operations ("supply chain department") as well as for supply chain executives and others who impact the supply chain.

The Central Role of the Supply Chain Department in CQO

Today, the supply chain department is becoming recognized as a multifaceted division within a hospital/health system that represents where cost, quality, and outcomes intersect. As noted previously (see Introduction, page 2), the hospital/health system supply chain consists of the following twelve focus areas:

- Continuous Process Improvement;
- Contracting;
- Data Management;
- Distribution;
- Education and Training;
- Internal Controls;
- Inventory Management;
- Purchasing;

---

[24] Greater New York Hospital Association, *GNYHA Summary of Major Provisions of the Patient Protection & Affordable Care Act & the Health Care and Education Reconciliation Act of 2010* (New York: GNYHA)

- Receiving;
- Reimbursement;
- Requisitioning;
- Value Analysis

Optimal performance in *each and every one* of these focus areas is essential to ensuring the successful operation of today's hospital/health system. In the current environment, the supply chain plays a critical strategic role in hospital/health system operations and is fundamental to achieving an organization's clinical and financial goals. Supply chain operations are generally thought to account for 30%–40% of a hospital's expenses, but this number typically reflects only the cost of goods. When other supply chain-related expenses (e.g., cost of procurement, storage, and time spent by clinicians and others on supply chain activities) are factored in, supply chain–related expenses can amount to as much as 50% of an organization's total budget.[25]

Among other key elements of supply chain performance, several areas are particularly important. For example, the centralization of procurement decisions has become vital because centralization supports efficient inventory management and volume-based purchasing, which leads to better pricing. Standardization, particularly in the area of physician/clinical preference items, is also critical when coupled with a robust evidence-based value analysis program that not only saves money but also positively affects quality and outcomes. Likewise, data collection and management are essential. Performance improvement throughout the organization—including the supply chain—hinges on accurate and timely data. Finally, supply chain-related technology is especially critical. State-of-the-art materials management information systems (MMIS) are essential for tracking the purchase and distribution of supplies, managing inventory levels, and so forth. For health systems, centralized procurement and accounts payable systems that all facil-

---

[25] Adapted from remarks by Jamie Kowalski in L. A. Jarousse, "Strategic Supply Chain Management," *Hospitals & Health Networks*, December 1, 2011. http://www.hhnmag.com/display/HHN-news-article.dhtml?d-crPath=/templatedata/HF_Common/NewsArticle/data/HHN/Magazine/2011/Dec/1211HHN_Feature_Gatefold.

ities within the system are required to use represent important ways for such systems to control costs and improve efficiencies. Additionally, if all systems are interfaced, key item data in the MMIS can and will flow into the clinical and financial systems, all leading to enterprise-wide data integrity.

The Ever-Broadening Skill Set Requirements for Supply Chain Executives

Today's environment also has important implications for supply chain executives' skill sets. Historically known as materials managers or purchasing directors, these executives' responsibilities traditionally focused on negotiating, ordering, receiving, and distributing medical/surgical supplies and equipment. The supply chain executive of today, however, is responsible for the total supply and logistics chain, which goes well beyond the procurement of medical/surgical supplies and equipment, instead to encompass the supply chain–related elements of other clinical and non-clinical areas such as food and nutrition services, biomedical engineering, laundry and linen, environmental services, plant operations, construction, capital equipment, and transportation/fleet services. Today's supply chain executives must have a deep understanding of all components of the supply chain; reimbursement policies, incentives, and penalties; evidence-based medicine; population health management; and so forth. They must build and maintain close working relationships with physicians, nurses, other clinicians, and virtually everyone involved in supply consumption and decision making, along with other key administrative departments such as finance and performance improvement. In the current environment, supply chain executives occupy a pivotal role that is critical to enabling a hospital/health system to provide the highest quality care in the most efficient and cost-effective manner possible. In short, today's supply chain executives are the organizational leaders who operate at the crucial intersection of cost, quality, and outcomes.

Attachment 1.

Major Milestones in Healthcare Reimbursement Policies [26, 27, 28]

DATE	DESCRIPTION
1929	The first hospital insurance plan in the United States was established by a group of employers in Dallas led by Baylor University. Considered the first Blue Cross plan in the United States, this plan was the foundation for the eventual establishment of Blue Cross and Blue Shield plans. Hospitals and physicians were reimbursed on a retrospective, cost-based, fee-for-service (FFS) basis.
1940s	Employers began offering health insurance as part of their employee benefits packages, launching the employer-based health insurance market. Under such plans, employers typically paid all or part of the premium costs. Hospitals continued to be paid on an FFS basis.
1965	Medicare and Medicaid programs were enacted by Congress providing health insurance coverage for Americans over the age of 65 and low-income Americans. Under these programs, retrospective, cost-based FFS reimbursement continued for hospitals.
1973	Congress passed the HMO Act, providing funding for the development of health maintenance organizations, which provide services to a specified population in a given geographic area for a fixed fee. This legislation marked the federal government's formal effort to promote healthcare delivery on a prepaid/capitated/managed care basis.
1982	Congress mandated the creation of a prospective payment system (PPS) for Medicare. This hospital payment system provides per-case reimbursement according to diagnosis-related groups (DRGs), a classification system that groups inpatient cases according to diagnosis. Under the DRG PPS, Medicare paid hospitals a flat rate per inpatient case based on diagnosis. PPS was designed to reward efficient hospitals and provide an incentive for inefficient hospitals to improve.
1998–2005	Congress enacted prospective payment systems for skilled nursing facilities (1998), home health agencies (1999), hospital-based outpatient services (2000), inpatient rehabilitation facilities (2002), and inpatient psychiatric facilities (2005).
2010	Congress enacted the Patient Protection and Affordable Care Act (ACA), which, in addition to its primary objective of providing health insurance coverage to uninsured/underinsured Americans, contains hospital-related reforms aimed at testing a variety of payment models such as accountable care organizations, patient-centered medical homes, shared savings programs, pay-for-performance programs, hospital value-based purchasing, and bundled care payments. The ACA also contains stiff penalties for unnecessary readmissions. These reforms signified a new era in hospital reimbursement, one in which reimbursement is directly tied to quality, outcomes, and patient care is delivered in the most efficient manner and setting.

---

[26] Green and Rowell, *Understanding Health Insurance*, Table 2-A (excerpts).
[27] *Medicare Hospital Prospective Payment System*, 7.
[28] Greater New York Hospital Association, *GNYHA Summary of Major Provisions*.

LEVEL I

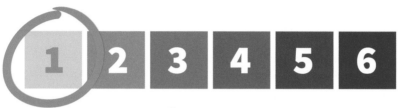

Overall Composite Score

Hospitals and health systems that score a composite rating of Level I on the Self-Assessment are operating across the board at the most basic level of supply chain management. In these organizations, the supply chain functions largely as a collection of component parts without a unifying plan to integrate the work and processes. In Level I organizations, the supply chain lacks a formal structure and an overarching strategy or vision linked to the larger strategy of the entire organization. The supply chain is *reactionary*—defined by and entrenched in practices that are rooted in the past (and with no foothold in the future)—with a focus that is primarily on day-to-day transactional operations and crisis management. It also typically operates with little or no awareness of or connection to changes occurring in the healthcare environment. As a consequence, it cannot or does not respond or adapt to the changing needs of the hospital/health system.

Level I hospitals/health systems are typically characterized by their independent and fractured approach to supply chain management. Supply chain activities are not centralized, and little collaboration exists between the supply chain components and clinicians/clinical departments or other administrative departments throughout the organization. Medical supplies and equipment are selected by individuals or departments without thorough vetting from a multidisciplinary team. Clinical and administrative departments and teams make purchasing and other supply chain–related decisions mostly in silos.

Because clinical and administrative departments tend to act independently, supply chain data are not routinely captured or tracked. The strategies employed by key supply chain components (e.g., purchasing, requisitioning, inventory, and contracting) are generally manual. There is no system to collect, connect, and integrate data. Systems and processes have not yet been established that allow for data sharing. Much of the accessible data are not available electronically and therefore cannot be analyzed or shared for process improvement purposes within or across departments.

The supply chain department's relationships with suppliers are confined to fairly simple transactions. The supply chain interacts and works with vendors to get an agreed-upon price on medical supplies and non-clinical items, but there is no mechanism or ability to work together with the goal of addressing supply chain issues that would streamline operations or optimize efficiencies.

At Level I, little attention is paid to staff education. Supply chain staff members learn "as they go." There is little to no formal training, onboarding, or mentorship programs to help employees acquire the knowledge, skills, and behaviors needed to become effective organizational team members.

In general, hospitals/health systems with supply chains rated at Level I reflect a culture that is transactional rather than strategic. Supply chain operations are rudimentary and underdeveloped. Activities that are essential to keep the supply chain moving get priority, but there is significant room for improvement in all categories of management and operations.

Level I: Performance by Focus Area

Continuous Process Improvement (CPI)

A supply chain–related CPI program is part of a larger strategy to identify and understand the best practices needed to drive significant improvements in hospital/health system operations. Because hospitals/health systems operating at Level I employ the most basic supply chain management systems and strategies, they typically do not include a CPI program. As a result, the organization's supply chain is focused on day-to-day operations and management and is not positioned to identify waste and inefficiency or support the organization's overall process improvement strategy.

Contracting

Contracting services at Level I are carried out by each hospital department individually rather than being centralized under the supply chain or within a group purchasing organization (GPO). Under this approach, each department chooses its own suppliers and preferred equipment. Thus, from an enterprise perspective, there is little ability to standardize products, manage inventory and costs, or achieve the kinds of economies of scale typically associated with volume-based purchasing.

Local contracts are often awarded in a "single-bid process," reflecting little or no consideration for overall cost to the institution or the possibility of saving money through a competitive bidding process. Simple, time-tested, traditional cost-effective strategies, such as a carefully prepared spreadsheet that compares each vendor's price/terms/cost to another's to determine the lowest qualified bid and improve the contracting process, are typically not used at this level.

Data Management

For hospitals/health systems operating at Level I, few data are collected, so data management is virtually nonexistent. Purchasing decisions are not supported by the organization's policies and procedures. There is no complete or actively

Item Master File
An institution's record of contracted and/or purchased items. The IMF typically includes contracted price, unit of measurement, vendor name, manufacturer name, vendor item number, catalog number, MMIS number, and units purchased.

maintained item master file (IMF); charges are not routinely captured; and data-based reports are not generated or available for supply chain, other administrative departments, and clinical departments to use in management and strategic planning. On the finance side, charges often are not captured, as they are manually documented, and billing data are frequently incomplete. Additionally, data do not flow among key departments due to inadequate systems.

Distribution

Organized and rapid distribution of medical supplies plays a pivotal role in assuring the efficacy of supply chain operations, and in some circumstances can be a matter of life and death. Without scheduled delivery dates and times, physicians, nurses, and other caregivers in all units must resort to guessing when critical supplies will be delivered or are forced to take time from patient care or other assigned responsibilities to secure necessary supplies. At Level I, supply distribution methods are at their most basic. Medical and non-medical supplies are distributed to clinical and support areas throughout the hospital/health system on an "as-needed" basis, and the hospital/health system does not adhere to a set distribution schedule. Supplies may not be delivered at all; instead, employees simply retrieve what they need from storerooms when they need it. Conversely, units may be significantly overstocked, which may result in expired products and waste.

Education and Training

No formal clinical or non-clinical supply chain–related education and training programs exist at Level I. There is no new hire orientation for supply chain employees; new staff members are trained "on the job." Training and education related to new products, equipment, or procedures are conducted informally as managers or supervisors see fit.

Internal Controls

When Sarbanes-Oxley ("SOX") was enacted in 2002, it mandated extensive internal review of financial procedures ("internal controls") for public entities and organizations receiving federal monies. Because hospitals/health systems receive federal dollars through Medicare and Medicaid, they are required to comply with SOX. While the integrity of financial systems is the principal focus of SOX, internal controls are critical to ensuring financial system integrity. Ideally, internal controls should focus on interactions both across hospital/health system departments and with suppliers. While some *informal* policies and procedures may exist in supply chain operations at Level I, there are no *formal* supply chain–related internal controls, policies, and procedures. Informal policies and procedures may or may not be adhered to or followed, resulting in uneven performance across the hospital/health system and putting the organization in regulatory jeopardy.

Inventory Management

Inventory management is rudimentary at Level I. Inventory is recorded neither manually nor digitally. Perpetual inventory (where the number of units of any inventory item and the total value of inventory can be obtained on any given day from the stock records) does not exist. As a result, the hospital/health system cannot keep a running balance of the number and/or cost of items, and routine measures such as cycle counting cannot be performed. Additionally, PAR levels are not established, thereby inhibiting the organization's ability to gauge when stock is getting low and needs replenishing.

Cycle Counting/Inventory
An inventory system where counts are performed continuously, often eliminating the need for an annual overall inventory. It is usually set up so that A items are counted regularly (i.e., every month), B items are counted semi-regularly (every quarter or six months), and C items are counted perhaps only once a year.

Without inventory controls, unvalued inventory is present across the enterprise. Patient items may get lost or go unaccounted for because there is no charge-to-order system. Inventory delivery systems have yet to be established, so no formal delivery process is documented or used, except perhaps for emergency situations. Due to the lack of inventory controls, clinical staff stockpiles product to prevent stock-outs.

Inventory gets turned on a limited basis with four or fewer active inventory turns in the hospital annually. In hospitals/health systems where inventory is not recorded and properly maintained, *more than 50%* of total inventory value is inactive. This affects the bottom line because the organization incurs a significant expense keeping those medical supplies and products on the books.

More than 1,000 stock-outs occur annually in hospitals/health systems, causing significant disruption to patient care, compromising patient safety, and affecting the entire organization's ability to deliver even basic healthcare and non- healthcare services.

Purchasing

The evolution of healthcare supply chain purchasing programs can be measured by the percentage of purchases conducted through an electronic data interchange (EDI) system. At Level I, the organization has yet to establish an EDI. Purchasing processes have also not evolved to the point of matching information on the invoice with information that backs up or supports the payment. The organization is not tracking the price and quantity of goods or services purchased, thereby increasing the probability that the hospital/health system is making overpayments, duplicating purchases, or, more seriously, not complying with government regulations.

Receiving

At Level I, there is no central receiving function for stock and non-stock purchases. Instead, such purchases are received by a number of locations across the hospital/health system. Vendors and distributors with their own fleet, as well as global carriers, deliver packages directly to the department or location that initiated the purchase.

Valued by some for its speed and simple delivery process, this approach compromises the organization's ability to accurately log and track items and ensure the right product gets to the right place at the right time. From a broader perspective, not having a centralized receiving process and/or warehouse can significantly complicate and affect security, traffic flow, and sometimes parking at these facilities.

Reimbursement

Level I-rated hospitals/health systems function without the infrastructure and/or information needed to accurately determine supply costs and/or reimbursement for supplies. Charge Description Master files contain information that is different from supply chain information and is reviewed independently of the supply chain. Typically, these organizations are characterized by a lack of coordination among such key operational areas as purchasing, contracting, storage, and distribution; manual data collection procedures; lack of a CPI program; inadequate data management practices; and other critical functions that form the foundation for optimal and appropriate reimbursement. Thus, reimbursement for Level I hospitals/health systems is haphazard, random, and unpredictable.

Requisitioning

At Level I, the compliance and supply chain departments have established a purchase requisition process to help manage requests for purchases as part of the organization's internal financial controls. However, all requisitions—regular, capital, service, etc.—are processed manually. At the department level, product requisitions are approved via an *ad hoc* process and established enterprise-wide policies are not enforced. Requests for goods and services are recorded and routed for approval within the hospital/health system by individual employees and then delivered to the finance department. Purchase requests are manually tracked and compared against internal departmental budgets and the general ledger.

Value Analysis

Hospitals and health systems operating at Level I reflect a culture that has not yet embraced value analysis. New products, services, and technology are introduced into units without undergoing a formal evaluation process whereby the cost and quality of the product and patient outcomes are all part of the conversation/dialogue and decision making. Instead of formal teams of clinicians and other subject matter experts, individuals and informal small groups make purchasing decisions on clinical preference items.

At Level I, supply chain activities receive minimal oversight from executives and tend to focus solely on lowest-cost purchasing activities. As a result, many, if not most, purchasing decisions are vendor-initiated and/or contract-driven. The checks and balances needed to support a healthy supply chain process are lacking.

Moreover, at Level I, cost is typically the primary decision driver for purchases, provision of services, and new technology adoption, and little to no consideration is given to how the item/service/technology affects patient safety, experience and outcome. Thus, data concerning quality and outcomes are not routinely captured and/or strategically used to analyze products, services, and technologies and inform purchasing decisions at the department, service line, or hospital/health system level.

Hospital Supply Chain Performance Self-Assessment™

LEVEL II

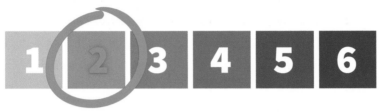

Overall Composite Score

Hospitals and health systems that score a composite rating of Level II on the Self-Assessment have begun to take important steps in the development of their supply chain but remain predominantly characterized by manual processes, limited data capture, largely decentralized operations, and departments working independently of one another with no formal strategy to share data and information. In many cases, established policies and procedures for supply chain operations exist, but they are not broadly communicated, followed, or enforced.

Level II hospitals/health systems still rely heavily on manual or rudimentary electronic processes. With few exceptions, supply chain activities are not coordinated centrally; however, where there is centralization (e.g., contracting), individual clinicians, departments, and service areas throughout the hospital/health system still have free license to negotiate directly with vendors and purchase off contract, severely limiting the advantages gained through centralization. While there is some awareness and even consensus that the hospital/health system would benefit from vetting its medical equipment and supply purchases through a multidisciplinary team comprising representatives from finance, supply chain, operations, and clinical staff, this typically does not occur. Moreover, formal value analysis is rudimentary, sporadic, and not carried out enterprise-wide.

The overarching issue facing Level II hospitals/health systems and affecting all operations is the absence of a well-articulated supply chain department strategy. Without this, the department cannot effectively align with other departments or the parent organization's strategy. In addition, supply chain data are not routinely captured or tracked, and there is no automated system that enables clinical data to be shared, analyzed, or synthesized with other key data. This affects the supply chain department administratively from a reporting and strategic planning perspective, and it also significantly influences the functions of contracting, purchasing, and inventory management. In effect, the lack of well-developed policies, procedures, and technological capability around data management affects supply chain operations on cost, quality, and outcomes measures.

The supply chain department's interactions with suppliers are principally driven by cost. Supply chain staff remain focused on trying to get the hospital/health system an agreed-upon price on medical supplies and non-clinical items. Clinicians typically have the closer relationship with vendors and distributors; therefore, vendors have little incentive to work collaboratively with supply chain management to address enterprise-wide supply chain operational issues.

Because the supply chain occupies a cross-disciplinary role within hospitals/health systems—often working across departments, administration, and clinical hierarchies—interdepartmental training and education are essential for sound supply chain management. In Level II organizations, there is minimal investment in education and training. There is no formal training or onboarding outside of the organization's new employee orientation. Supply chain staff is educated on the job, and non-supply chain staff gets no introduction or instruction regarding supply chain policies and operations.

Hospitals/health systems rated at Level II overall are operating at the low end of the CQO spectrum. There is substantial room for improvement in all areas of supply chain operations.

Level II: Performance by Focus Area

Continuous Process Improvement (CPI)

A supply chain–related CPI program should be tied to the overall hospital/ health system's strategy to identify and promote the practices that drive significant improvements in organizational operations. Similar to other areas in Level II hospitals/health systems, supply chain CPI processes, procedures, and technologies are instituted and implemented at half measure. They exist in some hospital/health system departments and service lines, but not in others. This variability weakens the organization, and opportunities for significant enhancements and advancement get overlooked. Instead of leading change, supply chain–related efforts tend to be reactionary at Level II.

Contracting

With a focus primarily on cost, little consideration is given to quality and outcomes measures in the contracting process at Level II. Contracting services are largely centralized, which is a significant step toward managing costs more effectively. Centralized buying opens the door to bulk purchasing, which strengthens the hospital's bargaining position and allows it to take advantage of quantity discounts. Consolidated orders reduce the transportation cost per unit, and the cost of order processing is substantially reduced due to fewer orders of larger quantities. However, Level II organizations still lack complete centralized contracting methodologies, which results in individuals and entire departments negotiating their own contracts with vendors of their choosing. As a result, multiple vendors exist for functionally similar products with limited rationale. The benefits of enterprise-wide product standardization are lost as a direct impact of this lax process.

The hospital/health system is affiliated with a national group purchasing organization (GPO) to leverage its buying power, yet the organization uses its GPO sporadically, operating on a case-by-case basis. At this level, the contracting process is not automatic or electronically activated, and the hospital/health system also does not utilize all the reporting tools available through the GPO. This, coupled with the fact that individual people and departments throughout the hospital/health system can do their own purchasing, makes it impossible to accurately track how much of the hospital/health system's spend is made on contract.

In addition to GPO contracts, local contracting is used occasionally, but often without the benefit of a competitive bidding process to garner the best price for products and services. The organization could strengthen its contracting service by putting in place and adhering to competitive bid policies and procedures.

Charge Description Master (CDM) or Chargemaster
The CDM is a master price list of supplies, devices, medications, services, procedures, and other items for which a distinct charge to the patient exists. It is a financial management tool that contains information about the organization's charges for the healthcare services it provides to patients. The CDM collects information on all the goods and services the organization provides to its patients.

Data Management

At Level II, data management is minimal. There is no IMF where inventory item records are created and policies for cost center expensing, replenishment, manufacturer, distributor, warehouse, and user-defined information about each item are stored and maintained. There *are* department-specific item listings, but these are updated rarely (if at all), making them essentially useless as the data become old and irrelevant.

Transactional data are routinely captured, and transactional reports are consistently generated and widely available. More complex data (point-in-time statistics and data sets used to identify trends) are not captured. This makes reporting capabilities quite limited, thereby affecting all other supply chain management areas. Absent widespread data capture, the supply chain is severely crippled, and CQO is difficult to achieve. Employees do not have the tools necessary to conduct value analysis and track reimbursements.

Supply charges are typically captured, but they are not recorded in a database or master file such as the CDM. Data elements such as charge descriptions, billing codes, pricing, etc., are not tracked; consequently, charges cannot be tied to the individual item file information or software applications that allow hospitals/health systems to integrate purchases and revenue cycle information.

Distribution

At this level, there is a set schedule for distributing medical and non-medical supplies to clinical and support areas, but the schedule is not adhered to and/ or is frequently out-of-date.

Without a reliable distribution system, hospital/health system employees feel forced to "bend the rules" and retrieve products from storerooms. With few inventory controls in place, these items often go unaccounted for. Enforcing the established distribution schedule will help the hospital/health system improve patient care and employee satisfaction and positively influence other supply chain operations, such as inventory, as well.

Education and Training

There is no established, ongoing formal clinical or non-clinical supply chain–related education and training program at Level II. Supply chain department employees and new staff are trained "on the job," with the exception of marginal training that occurs at new-hire orientation.

Any training and education related to new products, equipment, or department-specific policies and procedures happens informally and solely at the discretion of the employee's supervisor or department head.

Internal Controls

At Level II, internal controls are required throughout the hospital/health system and in each department, including the supply chain. The existence of internal controls and their enforcement/adherence throughout the hospital/ health system is a good barometer of how well the supply chain is functioning.

At this level, formal supply chain–related internal controls, policies, and procedures do exist, but there is no process or safeguard in place to ensure they are current. Because the supply chain department overlaps and interacts with so many other areas and departments within the hospital/health system, it needs to develop a control environment—a team of key individuals that determines safeguards and supports/enforces established processes. Core group participants should come from different areas of the supply chain such as logistics/transportation, purchasing, and warehouse/inventory, as well as from finance and human resources. Executive buy-in is crucial for setting expectations toward compliance throughout the organization.

Inventory Management

Inventory management is very basic at Level II, relying on a labor-intensive manual system rather than storing data and managing stock electronically. Inventory enterprise-wide is accounted for manually, requiring continuous monitoring to ensure that each transaction is recorded and that products are maintained at appropriate stocking levels. This approach makes it more difficult to share inventory information interdepartmentally and across the entire hospital/health system. The lack of computerization makes accessing inventory records a cumbersome process. It is neither cost-efficient nor quality-based because it translates to supply chain staff and clinical staff spending valuable time monitoring inventory levels, time that could be applied to more strategic supply chain activities or spent with a patient. Similarly, the charge-to-order system is also a manual process in Level II hospitals/health systems, requiring clinicians to use their time initiating a paper trail to process patient items.

PAR levels exist for major clinical areas but are only checked sporadically, significantly inhibiting the organization's ability to gauge when stock needs replenishing. Additionally, PAR levels are rarely used, and clinical or supply chain staffs use past knowledge or experience to determine reordering needs. As a result, department staff stockpiles product to make sure product is available when needed.

Cycle counting is performed on an "as-needed" basis, with no posted or established schedule. Additionally, cycle counting is performed without the benefit of ABC analysis, so there is no selective inventory control or prioritization of items considered of high value and very important to be kept in stock.

With few inventory controls and those in place only marginally enforced, unvalued inventory exists throughout the hospital/health system. Inventory is valued only in major departments (operating room, isolation room, catheter lab), and represents more than 75% of total inventory throughout the organization. Storerooms house high levels of inventory and carry a number of expired items. Some departments are stocked by the storeroom; others keep their own stock, leading to substantial accounting problems, uncertainty, confusion, and most importantly, valuable time lost in emergency situations.

Inventory gets turned on a limited basis. There are fewer than eight active inventory turns in the hospital annually. In Level II hospitals/health systems where inventory is typically neither recorded accurately nor routinely maintained, up to 50% of total inventory value is inactive inventory. With just a few additional inventory controls enacted and/or enforced, the organization could significantly reduce waste and increase efficiency.

Stock-outs can seriously compromise patient care and safety. Supply chains managing inventory operations from a CQO perspective are cognizant of these risks and institute controls to reduce or eliminate their occurrence. Up to 800 stock-outs occur annually in Level II organizations, providing ample opportunity for improvement in this area.

Purchasing

With respect to purchasing, Level II hospitals/health systems are still considered to be very basic. These organizations have established an EDI system, allowing for the electronic exchange of data between systems, but it is only used for medical, surgical, and laboratory items purchased through key distributors. At most, EDI is used for 35% of all purchase lines in the hospital/health system and represents approximately 10% of the total spend on purchases. Other purchases are placed via the buyers calling or faxing purchase orders to vendors, which results in a transactional supply chain.

To support the purchasing function, processes are in place to match information on the purchase order to the receipt and the invoice; however, these processes are used sporadically and typically only when there is a payment issue with a vendor (or when some other red flag indicates a problem). Three-way price/quantity matching (P.O.→receipt→invoice) is performed manually, requiring staff time to track down information that supports the payment. The organization's spotty and unpredictable data capture and management significantly affects this aspect of purchasing. Without consistent tracking of the price and quantity of goods or services purchased, it is difficult to conduct a three-way match, with or without an EDI system.

Receiving

At this level, the receiving function is centralized but still a manual operation. Stock purchases are received at the loading dock and then logged and tracked to the department or location that initiated the purchase, leaving a paper trail.

There is a centralized process in place for receiving non-stock purchases as well, but adherence to the practice by departments and service lines is erratic and sporadic. These items, while not stock items, still must be accounted for and tracked as they are hospital/health system property for record-keeping purchases. The organization's uneven enforcement of its centralized receiving process can result in lost inventory and significantly affect the organization's bottom line.

Reimbursement

Level II hospitals/health systems use supply-related cost and revenue metrics to evaluate their performance against available benchmarks for high-level purposes, such as total supply chain budget and labor costs, but their limited use of automation and inconsistent data capture puts finer analyses out of reach. There are no strategies or internal controls targeting the collection and manipulation of essential data that would help the organization see purchasing trends and how they affect clinical outcomes and financial reimbursement.

Requisitioning

Healthcare organizations operating at Level II have established an enterprise-wide electronic requisitioning system to manage requests for purchases, but it is seldom used. Generally, electronic requisitioning represents only 5% of all purchase lines and 5% of the organization's total spend. The remaining requests for goods and services are processed manually, with each department tracking and comparing its purchase requests against budget, governed by its own approval structure and process.

Value Analysis

Hospitals/health systems operating at Level II recognize and acknowledge the need for value analysis in their organizations but have not yet implemented a formal value analysis program. Supply chain, finance, operations, and clinical staff typically make purchasing decisions in isolation. New clinical and non-clinical products, services, and technology are subject to department-specific evaluation; each group conducts its own analysis to determine value, and new initiatives result from clinical or physician-driven requests for new or replacement products. While this "silo approach" may seem more efficient in the short run, it rarely benefits the organization in the long run because it often results in overpriced and duplicated products, unusable equipment, overstock, and finger-pointing.

Executive leadership provides direction on cost reduction and other supply chain–related initiatives only for major acquisitions and purchases, leaving very little oversight or accountability for other purchases. Cost reduction on medical/surgical products is typically driven by the expiration of existing contracts or new product needs.

There are occasional instances and indications of a holistic CQO approach when assessing new products and services at Level II, but cost is still the primary decision driver for most purchases. Clinical data, outcomes, and reimbursement levels have some bearing on the evaluation process for certain initiatives at the department or service-line level, but one rarely sees the fully integrated CQO approach. Work is usually carried out in silos across the hospital/health system, with very little interdepartmental communication and data-sharing. Typically, supply chain staff, clinicians, and finance staff focus on cost, clinical, and reimbursement/financial outcome data, respectively, because these are the data they "own."

LEVEL III

Overall Composite Score

Hospitals and health systems scoring a composite rating of Level III on the Self-Assessment are organizations that still employ outdated practices but are actively striving to update them. The supply chain team has implemented select strategies and invested in some of the necessary infrastructure to move the organization toward a more holistic approach to supply chain management, but significantly more remains to be done before the supply chain is functioning optimally. Limited use of technology and automation and the lack of standardization and enforcement of internal controls keep the department from realizing its full potential.

Level III supply chain operations are predominantly characterized by a hybrid of automated and manual processes, limited data capture and reporting functions, partially centralized operations, and departments that work independently of one another. In many cases, the organization has established the infrastructure it needs to support solid supply chain management, but the lack of internal controls and the failure to employ CPI methodologies in all departments and service lines cripple its efforts toward migrating to a more holistic CQO approach.

There *are* established policies and procedures for supply chain functions in most areas, but they are followed sporadically and are erratically enforced. Contracting, purchasing, and value analysis activities generally are conducted in silos rather than through a coordinated approach to driving down costs and integrating cost with quality and outcomes measures. At this level, the supply chain department's efforts are still principally transactional, with the department continuing to function more as an enabler that supports daily operations than as a leader.

In an era where data are increasingly considered "king," and evidence-based healthcare practices are not only the trend but also directly tied to reimbursement, sound data management is paramount. This area provides the supply chain's greatest opportunity for growth and impact within the hospital/health system. Greater data capture and oversight to ensure that technology and procedures are used consistently will provide the foundational building blocks for CQO. The supply chain department can begin integrating quality and outcomes data with cost data to work across department lines and influence decision making.

Group Purchasing Organization (GPO)
An organization that negotiates volume discount contracts with suppliers on behalf of its member facilities, providing them with favorable pricing, terms and conditions, and other benefits. GPO participants can include hospitals, medical group practices, nursing homes and other long-term care facilities, surgery centers, managed care organizations, home infusion providers, provider pharmacies, clinics, and integrated delivery networks.

Investments in technology and systems integration, along with education and training, will also strengthen and improve supply chain operations. Level III hospitals/health systems have an IMF and CDM; they use EDI; and they employ an MMIS and computerized point-of-use and enterprise asset management systems. However, these valuable tools and technologies are underused. Hospital/health system employees are not routinely trained on these systems; the technology and practices have not been applied and implemented throughout the organization. Too often, active use of these tools is limited to just a few departments and/or service lines.

Overall, Level III hospitals/health systems are operating on the middle to low end of the CQO spectrum. Supply chain management is focused on cost and has yet to fully embrace and integrate quality and outcomes into operations. However, the opportunity exists, with policies and procedures in place, the supply chain department's presence in clinical departments established, and reimbursement a significant focus.

Level III: Performance by Focus Area

Continuous Process Improvement (CPI)

CPI methodologies are applied to supply chain functions in Level III hospitals/health systems; however, CPI processes, procedures, and technology are standardized only within individual departments and/or service lines. A strong CPI program affects all aspects of supply chain management and is crucial to making the transition to a CQO approach. Standardization across the enterprise is necessary for the organization to streamline operations and gain efficiencies in supply chain functionality.

Contracting

At Level III, contracting services are partially centralized, but individuals and departments still negotiate their own contracts with suppliers, which weakens the organization's bargaining position. Less than 25% of the organization's spend is contracted, so even though the supply chain department may have negotiated good contracts with many of the institution's suppliers, many employees go outside those contracts for their purchases. Every time they do, they most likely pay a higher price. Unmanaged spending, often without purchase orders, points to larger control and accounting issues. With more than 75% of the hospital/health system's expenditures falling into this category, cost-saving measures, such as enterprise-wide product standardization, can't be implemented, leading to wasteful spending.

The hospital/health system is affiliated with one or more GPOs to leverage buying power, yet the organization uses its GPO options less than 50% of the time. As a result, the organization is not taking full advantage of the pricing it can obtain through a GPO portfolio.

The hospital/health system uses local contracting through a competitive bidding process, but only for major projects, and the process focuses only on cost. The organization could strengthen its local contracting efforts by competitively bidding all contracts and requiring that the bids take into account total costs, patient safety, and clinical outcomes, as appropriate.

Data Management

Data management at Level III can best be described as fundamentally basic—structured, but with minimal maintenance and upkeep. Inventory item records exist for many items, and user-defined information about each item is stored in the IMF, but the files are marginally managed and poorly maintained. Updates occur less than quarterly, and/or multiple FTEs have the ability to add, change, or update items. However, with the IMF framework and maintenance policies in place, the organization is in a good position to significantly improve data management and bring value to the process.

Transactional data and static point-in-time statistics are routinely captured and reported widely. More complex data that would allow for internal and external trend reporting are not captured, limiting the hospital/health system's evolution to a true CQO approach and affecting all other areas of supply chain management. Without extensive data capture, advanced analyses cannot occur. This makes it difficult for the supply chain department to generate the information needed to influence clinicians and hospital administration to make changes that will lower cost, improve patient safety and reimbursement levels, and reduce penalties associated with poor clinical outcomes.

Like other aspects of data management, a structure exists for capturing supply charges, but maintenance is low. Level III organizations have a minimally maintained CDM, so data elements, such as charge descriptions, billing codes, and pricing, can be tracked and recorded. Charges are rarely tied to the individual item file information; purchases and revenue cycle information are not integrated.

Distribution

In Level III hospitals/health systems, a set supply distribution schedule exists, but its enforcement tends to be very lax. The schedule is seldom updated and is adhered to only sporadically.

Distribution is key to getting the "right product to the right place at the right time." This function, if well managed, could create goodwill with clinicians and staff. When it is poorly managed, frustrations rise quickly and employees feel forced to work outside of the rules. By examining its supply distribution schedule for any weak links, as well as making distribution and adherence to the set schedule a supply chain priority, Level III organizations can easily improve employee satisfaction, contribute to patient safety, and build trust with other departments.

Education and Training

Level III hospitals/health systems conduct formal (clinical or non-clinical) supply chain–related education and training programs at least once a year. Training and education related to new products, equipment, and technology generally occur informally and at the discretion of the employee's supervisor or department head. With the exception of new employee orientation and randomly held trainings, supply chain department employees and hospital/health system staff are trained "on the job" with regard to supply chain practices.

Because the supply chain crosses institutional silos more frequently than any other department, education and training are particularly important. The organization should strive toward establishing formal clinical *and* non-clinical supply chain-related education and training on a routine, ongoing basis, offering a program fully integrated throughout the entire enterprise.

Internal Controls

Internal controls are essential to building and maintaining a robust, successful healthcare supply chain. Without these checks and balances, the supply chain cannot deliver a performance that supports a CQO approach.

Level III hospitals/health systems have established formal supply chain-related internal controls. There are written supply chain policies and procedures applicable to supply chain functions that touch departments throughout the organization, but controls ensuring that the policies and procedures are current and being used enterprise-wide are not being implemented. Internal controls—including all supply chain policies and procedures—are reviewed and updated only sporadically and are not adhered to consistently.

Best practices call for regular reviews of policies and procedures as well as periodic audits to ensure compliance. Without these, the supply chain's efficiency is compromised and its full value unrealized.

Inventory Management

Level III hospitals/health systems employ a perpetual inventory system for the hospital/health system storeroom, allowing for real-time tracking of item use as well as inventory levels for individual items. Computerized point-of-use and enterprise asset management systems allow the department to provide a highly detailed view of changes in storeroom inventory and make it possible to provide immediate reporting of the amount of inventory in stock and accurately reflect the number of products on hand. However, perpetual inventory does not exist for other inventory areas such as nursing units, the operating room, radiology, and the cath lab. At these locations, inventory is maintained manually, requiring tight controls and strong vigilance to ensure each transaction is recorded and that inventory remains adequately stocked. This places Level III organizations on the lower end of the CQO spectrum regarding inventory management, as stock-outs inevitably occur, and clinicians spend precious time tracking down necessary items, potentially compromising patient care and safety. In some cases, it may affect financial outcomes as well, as reimbursement becomes more related to patient outcomes.

PAR levels exist for all clinical areas but are only checked sporadically, perhaps less than once each year, making it difficult to gauge whether levels are set too high or too low, contributing to stock-outs or overinvestment in product inventory. Clinical staff remains concerned about having inventory when needed, and as a result, stockpiles product.

Cycle counts to verify inventory accuracy are executed periodically but irregularly. While cycle counts do take place, there is no established schedule. Furthermore, cycle counting is performed without the benefit of ABC analysis, so there is no selective inventory control or prioritization of crucial inventory items and those that are considered "high value."

In keeping with other areas of Level III hospital/health system operations, some aspects of inventory management are computerized and consistent, while others remain manual and inconsistent. For instance, Level III organizations have charge-to-order systems, but they are used to process no more than 50% of patient items. Best practices indicate that *at least* 90% of all items used enterprise-wide should be on a charge-to-order system. While the technology is in place for these organizations, its use must increase to directly affect revenue capture.

With sporadic cycle counts and poor oversight of PAR levels, unvalued inventory exists widely throughout the hospital/health system. In any department or location, more than 50% but less than 75% of inventory is unvalued.

The storeroom stocks all hospital departments instead of using a low-unit-of-measure distribution (LUM) program in departments or a Just-in-Time (JIT) system. There are controlled levels of inventory in the hospital storeroom, however, and few to no expired items.

Inventory gets turned on a limited basis. There are 9–12 active inventory turns in the hospital/health system annually. In Level III hospitals/health systems, where only the main storeroom has perpetual inventory and all inventory is sporadically maintained, inactive inventory represents up to 40% of total inventory value.

Up to 600 stock-outs occur annually in Level III organizations, placing them on the lower end of the CQO spectrum. With just a few additional inventory controls enacted and/or enforced, the organization could significantly reduce waste and increase efficiency through its inventory management processes.

Low Unit of Measure (LUM) Distribution

In contrast to the traditional bulk model of shipping inventory in full-case quantities to hospital storerooms and subsequently to patient care areas, low-unit-of-measure (LUM) or best-unit-of-measure (BUM) involves breaking cases into smaller units, which are delivered directly to patient areas.[1]

Purchasing

Level III hospitals/health systems use EDI for most items purchased through the prime distributor—medical, surgical, laboratory, etc.—and up to 25% of all other items purchased. EDI is used for up to 45% of all purchase lines in the hospital/health system and represents approximately 20% of the total purchased spend.

While having an EDI system is crucial to supply chain management from a CQO perspective, the low level of adoption and usage still puts Level III hospitals/health systems on the lower end of the CQO spectrum. Relying on manual processes exposes the organization to data entry errors, discrepancies, and misinterpretations, and significantly impedes supply chain activities across the board. Hospitals/health systems with purchasing programs rated at Level III typically experience higher inventory levels, higher error rates, slower delivery and distribution times, and a poorer capacity for product planning and forecasting than those using EDI more broadly.

There is electronic three-way price/quantity matching (P.O.→receipt→invoice) to support the purchasing function, but the option is only used with selected vendors and certain items and represents less than 35% of all purchase lines and only 10% of total spend purchased. The organization's contracting policies and limited data management impede making full use of the EDI system. With departments purchasing many of their items independently and off contract with only sporadic maintenance and updates to the IMF and CDM, EDI and reporting value is compromised.

Receiving

The receiving function in Level III hospitals/health systems is centralized and computerized. There is an MMIS; however, loading information into it is still a manual operation. Stock purchases are received at the loading dock and then logged into the MMIS by hand, whereby they can be tracked to the department or location that initiated the purchase.

A centralized process is in place for receiving non-stock purchases as well. At least 25% of all hospital/health system departments and service lines adhere to the organization's non-stock receiving policies and procedures. By tightening up central receiving efforts, the hospital/health system can more easily keep track of its property and manage its inventory.

Reimbursement

Reimbursement is central to the CQO equation. Level III hospitals/health systems use supply-related cost and revenue metrics to evaluate their performance against available benchmarks in major areas like total supply chain budget and labor costs, but only select departments use these measures to evaluate their performance on a regular basis. This places Level III organizations on the lower end of the CQO spectrum.

The supply chain department's policies, procedures, and performance in other areas of supply chain management have great bearing here, as limited data capture and reporting tools, loose controls, inconsistent enforcement, and unreliable inventory procedures affect the organization's ability to measure with confidence and provide accurate data for reimbursement purposes.

Automation of many supply chain processes, tightening controls, and integrating existing technology throughout the entire enterprise is critical to building the organization's performance, particularly from a financial perspective.

Requisitioning

Healthcare organizations operating at Level III have established an enterprise-wide electronic requisitioning system to manage requests for purchases, but they could benefit from using the system more widely. Electronic requisitioning is used by at least 25% of key departments for all requests throughout the hospital/health system (including capital and service requests as well as requests for information), and represents at least 15% of all purchase lines and 10% of the total spend purchased by the organization.

The remaining requests for goods and services are processed manually, with each department tracking and comparing its own purchase requests against budget, governed by its own approval structure and process.

Value Analysis

A Level III hospital/health system has an active value analysis program, but the program itself remains segmented by departmental lines, with operations and clinical staff focused on quality and clinical outcomes and the finance and supply chain departments focused primarily on cost. While some interdepartmental communication and collaboration exists, the hospital/health system culture still reflects a predominantly siloed approach to value analysis.

Supply chain leadership evaluates major purchases for cost and includes clinical evaluations. Yet fewer than 25% of new products, services, and technology are evaluated by an interdepartmental team prior to purchase, leaving 75% of the hospital/health system spend to individual departments and the influence of controlling interests. This unbalanced practice translates to narrow executive oversight, limited accountability, and discord and infighting between divisions within the hospital/health system, while perpetuating a culture of separateness and mistrust.

The CQO model has been somewhat embraced and partially integrated when assessing new products and services at the department and service line level in Level III hospitals/health systems, but cost is still the primary decision driver for most supply purchases. Clinical data and reimbursement levels come to bear more often in the evaluation process for specific clinical initiatives. Supply chain managers still chiefly "own" cost, clinical staff "owns" clinical/quality data, and finance "owns" financial outcomes and reimbursement. In these organizations, the supply chain department recognizes the valuable role it can play in CQO, and some inroads have been made toward that end, but there is much room for improvement in raising awareness and education as well as building relationships with essential players in the organization.

LEVEL IV

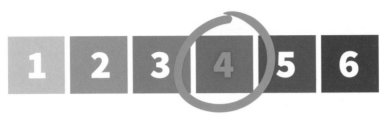

Overall Composite Score

Hospitals/health systems with a Level IV composite score have a strategic outlook that acknowledges CQO as fundamental to optimal success. They have laid the groundwork to approach supply chain management from the *intersection* of CQO but have yet to fully realize their vision.

Key elements for success are in place—the infrastructure and technology exists, internal controls are established, and interdisciplinary teams have been identified to work together to detect and resolve issues that compromise patient care and affect the bottom line—however, the organization does not make full use of the technology, policies, and processes it has developed for supply chain to operate strategically from the CQO intersection.

The hospital/health system uses its technology at approximately half capacity. Data capture related to contracting, purchasing, requisitioning, and inventory control is partial and incomplete, with only certain departments and service lines using the sophisticated electronic and automated systems available, and then only some of the time. The data that *are* captured are not consistently maintained. Similar patterns can be seen regarding internal controls (including supply chain policies and procedures); they exist, but are adhered to and enforced only sporadically. Processes, procedures, and technology are standardized across at least 50% of hospital/health system departments and/or service lines.

At Level IV, the supply chain department leads cost reduction and other supply chain–related initiatives with physician involvement, and there is significant integration between cost-, quality-, and outcomes-driven initiatives at the department, service line, or hospital/health system level, but not enterprise-wide integration. Supply chain operations are more automated than not, and most data capture is electronic, although manual practices and processes still occur.

The organization offers formal clinical and non-clinical supply chain–related education and training at least annually. The supply chain department works closely with multidisciplinary teams throughout the hospital/health system, but their efforts are primarily focused on high-level/select clinical operations. As a result, an interdepartmental committee evaluates fewer than half (25%–50%) of new products, services, and technology prior to purchase.

The greatest challenges Level IV hospitals/health systems face are tied to implementation and enforcement. The organization has the basic infrastructure it needs to support supply chain management with a more holistic CQO approach, but it has not developed the discipline and practices needed to flourish. In healthcare organizations with Level IV operations, the supply chain department is emerging as a valuable and indispensable resource. With stronger emphasis on collaboration, data management, and process improvement methods, the department will become less transactional, more strategic, and increasingly important to the institution's overall success.

Level IV: Performance by Focus Area

Continuous Process Improvement (CPI)

In an ongoing effort to drive process improvements enterprise-wide, CPI methodologies are applied to supply chain functions and standardized across at least 50% of the hospital/health system's departments and/or service lines. Some of these efforts are supply chain–centric, though most require significant collaboration and a multidisciplinary approach. At Level IV, CPI is implemented in small and large ways—some process improvements take place incrementally over time, while others require major change initiatives.

Supply chain leaders reflect a commitment to improvement, and CPI has become part of the ethos of the department. As the department becomes more strategic in its focus, it will apply CPI to supply chain functions increasingly throughout the hospital/health system.

Contracting

At Level IV, contracting services are partially centralized, but the organization has plans actively under development to centralize contracting enterprise-wide. While the supply chain department is working with departments and units across the organization to increase efficiency, streamline spend, and reduce duplication of common activities across projects, a significant number of individuals, units, and departments are still negotiating and managing their own contracts. Ineffective management and governance of supplier contracts affects hospitals negatively in the way of missed savings opportunities, revenue loss, and waste.

Between 25% and 50% of the organization's spend is contracted. Without integrated systems and a single repository to manage contracts and processes, contracting services at this level are not hitting cost measures and are completely unable to address quality concerns and outcomes. With 50%–75% of the organization's spend off-contract and therefore much harder to track and control, the institution has considerable room to strengthen and improve contracting services.

The hospital/health system is affiliated with a national GPO to leverage its buying power and may utilize a local group aggregation GPO for contract pricing and electronic activation for at least 50% of product purchases. The hospital/health system is not taking full advantage of its GPO membership(s) as it is not implementing all the reporting, benchmarking, templates, and tools that GPOs offer their members. When only partial use is made of the full range of GPO solutions, typically the supply chain department focuses almost exclusively on cost, and therefore is not looking at contracting/supply chain management from the more holistic CQO perspective.

Some GPO contract categories are locally negotiated. The hospital/health system uses a competitive bidding process in its local contracting efforts, but the process focuses solely on cost and does not take into account quality and outcomes measures. The organization could strengthen its contracting service by requiring that, in addition to cost, bids for local contracts include patient safety, clinical outcomes, and reimbursement data.

Data Management

Perhaps no area is as fundamental to managing the supply chain from the intersection of cost, quality, and outcomes as data management. Without valid, consistent, and reliable data, the supply chain department simply does not have the information needed to make sound decisions and interact knowledgeably with colleagues throughout the hospital/health system. Level IV organizations are characterized by having one IMF into which multiple item files have been updated and transitioned; however, it is only sporadically maintained. Having one consolidated IMF is an important step toward a more advanced supply chain operation; failing to update it regularly severely limits the organization's growth from a CQO perspective.

Charges are captured in the CDM, but like the IMF, no reliable schedule for its maintenance exists. The CDM is updated less than quarterly. At Level IV, the hospital/health system typically does not have an automated CDM tool that standardizes pricing and descriptions for line items and monitors for regulatory compliance. There may be a documented process and policy in place regarding manual updates, but the process is not routinely followed. Reports that indicate trends and reveal variances are used periodically throughout the hospital/health system to make evidence-based decisions regarding contracting, purchasing, and policies relating to item use.

Collectively, these data management practices place Level IV hospitals/ health systems in the middle range of the CQO spectrum.

Distribution

Level IV hospitals/health systems have a set distribution schedule for distributing patient care–related supplies within the hospital/health system. The schedule is posted and updated regularly, but it is adhered to only for critical clinical areas. Departments and units outside of these areas cannot rely on the distribution schedule for their supply deliveries. This shortcoming undermines confidence in the supply chain department, encourages staff to work "outside the system" to get what they need, and works against the overall strategies and goals the supply chain department has established and strives to achieve through its policies and procedures.

Education and Training

Level IV organizations regard ongoing education and training as an important supply chain strategy and have established formal clinical *and* non-clinical education and training for staff. Formal training programs are offered at least once each year. Employees are primarily trained "on the job" regarding supply chain practices; however, supply chain policies and procedures are in place for most essential functions.

As the supply chain department continues to focus on CQO, fosters collaborations with physicians and other clinical staff, and seeks to bridge institutional silos, supply chain education grows in importance. Supply chain education offered on an ongoing basis, fully integrated throughout the entire institution, will help the department demonstrate its strategic value.

Internal Controls

Level IV hospitals/health systems rate mid-range on the CQO spectrum regarding internal controls. Policies and procedures for supply chain functions pertaining to all departments and units throughout the organization have been established and are reviewed and updated annually, but they are not adhered to consistently. The organization conducts an internal audit to "catch" issues like poor compliance; however, the audit is conducted less than once every three years. Consequently, many issues are overlooked for long periods of time, and supply chain performance suffers.

Inventory Management

Hospitals/health systems operating at Level IV use computerized point-of-use and enterprise asset management systems to provide a highly detailed view of inventory changes in the organization's storeroom and nursing units, but not for other major inventory areas.

Electronic Health Record (EHR)
A computer-accessible, interoperable resource of clinical and administrative information pertinent to the health of an individual. Information drawn from multiple clinical and administrative sources is used primarily by a broad spectrum of clinical personnel involved in the individual's care, enabling them to deliver and coordinate care and promote wellness.

The hospital/health system uses a perpetual inventory system for the storeroom and nursing units. Items are tracked in real time, and the system reflects current inventory levels for each item. However, even when using a sophisticated perpetual inventory management system, the hospital/health system must still conduct proper maintenance, including manual inventory counts. Scanned data tell the supply chain department exactly what inventory *should be* on hand. The manual inventory count *confirms* these data and helps the department determine how much inventory has been lost, stolen, or is past its "use by" date. The organization does well with conducting routine maintenance in the storeroom, but it does not maintain its nursing units consistently.

The hospital/health system uses a manual inventory process for other major inventory areas (operating room, radiology, cath lab, etc.), relying on employees to record each transaction to ensure inventory remains adequately stocked. This places Level IV organizations mid-range on the CQO spectrum, as stock-outs are prone to occur, potentially jeopardizing patient care and safety.

PAR levels exist for all clinical areas. The numbers are reviewed at least annually, and performance by area is reported to clinical operations leadership. Cycle counting to verify inventory accuracy is also executed annually based on ABC analysis, which prioritizes crucial inventory items and those considered high value.

Level IV hospitals/health systems use an electronic charge-to-order system to process between 50% and 75% of all patient items. This system is an important tool from a CQO perspective; in addition to inventory control, it aids the supply chain department in revenue capture. It also provides patient data to be used in future analyses, and, if interfaces are established, flows directly into the electronic health record (EHR). With modest effort in this area, the supply chain department could increase its performance to meet the standard for best practices—that is, *at least* 90% of all patient items used enterprise-wide would be on a charge-to-order system.

Even with using inventory controls such as cycle counts and PAR level review, unvalued inventory is still widespread. In any department or location, more than 25% but less than 50% of inventory is unvalued.

The hospital/health system storeroom houses and delivers emergency stock. Individual departments and units within the hospital/health system are stocked using a LUM program. Products are picked and packed for a department PAR level in the lowest unit-of-measure—typically "each" or "box"—streamlining supply chain activities and facilitating item delivery to end users within the healthcare facility.

Inventory gets turned on a fairly regular basis with more than twelve active inventory turns annually. Although the hospital/health system uses a perpetual inventory system and LUM program, inactive inventory represents up to 30% of total inventory value. Extending perpetual inventory practices to all departments and units and conducting routine (manual) inventory maintenance enterprise-wide will help the supply chain department lower that number significantly.

Up to 400 stock-outs occur throughout the hospital annually for Level IV hospitals/health systems, again placing them in the mid-range on the

> **Electronic Data Interchange (EDI)**
> Intercompany, computer-to-computer transmission of business information in a standard format. For EDI purists, "computer to computer" means direct transmission from the originating application program to the receiving or processing application program. An EDI transmission consists only of business data, not any accompanying verbiage or free-form messages. Purists might also contend that a standard format is one that is approved by a national or international standards organization, as opposed to formats developed by industry groups or companies.

CQO spectrum. Tighter inventory controls will strengthen the overall inventory management process and help the organization achieve performance more in line with best practices for stock-outs—namely, fewer than 100 per year.

Purchasing

Purchasing activities at Level IV are largely streamlined for most items that the hospital/health system secures through its prime distributors. The organization uses an EDI system for medical, surgical, and laboratory supplies and up to 35% of all other items purchased system-wide. EDI is used for up to 55% of all purchase lines and represents approximately 40% of the total spend purchased by the organization.

EDI is an essential business practice for hospital/health system supply chains wanting to operate from the intersection of cost, quality, and outcomes. Hospitals/health systems rated at Level IV in purchasing could significantly improve productivity, accuracy, and efficiency levels by increasing EDI usage. Making full use of the hospital's EDI system benefits the supply chain in multiple ways; it allows for real-time transactional analysis, eliminates human error, improves forecasting, and allows the organization to carry lower inventory levels. Additionally, using EDI and electronic systems helps transition the supply chain to a more strategic model.

To support the purchasing function, there is electronic three-way price/quantity matching (P.O.→receipt→invoice) for all vendors and/or items. This system is used for up to 50% of all purchase lines and represents 35% of total spend purchased.

Receiving

The receiving function for stock purchases in Level IV hospitals/health systems is centralized. Employees use a handheld device to enter some of these purchases into the MMIS, and others are entered manually.

A centralized process is in place for receiving non-stock purchases. At least half of all hospital/health system departments and service lines adhere to the organization's non-stock receiving policies and procedures.

Up to 50% of departments and service lines bypass the organization's receiving policies and procedures. This makes the hospital/health system vulnerable to theft and fraud and complicates the supply chain department's ability to adequately track products and account for inventory.

Reimbursement

Metrics link operational performance to the hospital/health system's strategy and allow supply chain executives to demonstrate the supply chain's contribution to the organization's overall business objectives. Hospitals/health systems operating at Level IV make high-level supply cost/revenue metrics and basic dashboards available for such purposes. While the capability exists to develop dashboards and sophisticated reports, the department's marginal data management performance significantly affects its ability to supply accurate and relevant data for reimbursement purposes.

From the supply chain perspective, improving reimbursement hinges on such efforts as tightening inventory controls, strengthening overall internal controls, enforcing policies and procedures relating to the IMF and CDM, etc. When this occurs, the critical role the supply chain department plays in the reimbursement arena will be firmly established.

Requisitioning

Level IV healthcare organizations have established an enterprise-wide electronic requisitioning system to manage requests for purchases. It is used by at least half of the hospital/health system's departments and service lines for all requests throughout the enterprise (including regular, capital, service, etc.), and represents up to 35% of all purchase lines and 30% of the total spend purchased by the organization.

The remaining requests for goods and services are not handled through the electronic requisitioning system, but by each hospital/health system department managing its own paper requests, which is regulated by that department's budget and approval procedure.

Value Analysis

Hospitals/health systems with Level IV value analysis programs reflect a culture that has partially embraced the CQO model. Supply chain is partially integrated with clinical operations, focusing on a number of select procedures and service lines, but not all. With these chosen few, supply chain staff works closely with clinicians to consider cost and quality issues, such as patient safety and clinical outcomes, as well as the potential ramifications regarding reimbursement when jointly making purchasing decisions for the hospital/health system.

The supply chain department provides direction around cost-reduction efforts and other supply chain–related initiatives with input from physicians. While there is shared ownership of the value analysis process at Level IV, the supply chain department has started to step into more of a leadership role. Where physicians bring a wealth of knowledge and expertise from a clinical perspective, and the finance department supplies data on reimbursement and financial outcomes, the supply chain department has started to own the *intersection* where interests merge and cost, quality, and outcomes coincide.

There is an established process for the introduction and adoption of new clinical and non-clinical products, services, and technologies. At this more advanced level of supply chain management, an interdepartmental committee comprising supply chain staff, clinicians, and employees relevant to the procedure or service line evaluates between 25% and 50% of new products.

There are signs of significant integration between cost-, quality-, and outcomes-driven initiatives at the department and service line as well as in some cases at the hospital/health system level. CQO has *started* to infiltrate the ethos and philosophy of the organization, but the permeation is not yet enterprise-wide. Evidence-based practices are common, and multidisciplinary teams are increasingly engaged to review processes and procedures to ensure the patient remains at the center of all decision making.

LEVEL V

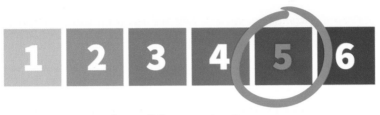

Overall Composite Score

Hospitals/health systems with a Level V composite score on the Self-Assessment are strategic and grounded in the fundamentals of the CQO approach to supply chain management. The supply chain department's vision ties to its parent healthcare organization's overall strategic goals while steadily working on putting the systems, policies, and personnel into place to take the institution from good to great. It is evolving from the traditional focus on cost to building a more comprehensive patient-centered model of supply chain management that factors in quality measures (e.g., patient safety and clinical outcomes) as well as financial outcomes and reimbursement into its decision making.

An interdisciplinary culture supports the integration of the supply chain and cost reduction throughout the hospital/health system. The supply chain department is almost fully integrated with the organization's clinical operations, crossing department lines to collaborate with clinicians and administrators from finance, quality improvement, and other departments to drive down costs and improve patient safety. Although the culture of cooperation and teamwork is dominant and pervasive, sporadic enforcement and varied levels of implementation of supply chain policies, procedures, and technologies leave room for growth in several areas.

Level V hospitals/health systems value the supply chain and have invested in the infrastructure and technology to support a robust operation internally and externally. Most procedures and activities are automated, streamlining operations and significantly reducing the margin of error commonly associated with many supply chain functions.

Data capture is widespread, and data are used to provide comprehensive analytics and sophisticated reports—but only sometimes. In short, the data exist, but they're not always used well or consistently. Hospitals/health systems operating at this level are fairly consistently gathering, tracking, and measuring data. The challenge isn't in acquiring or accessing data, but in using and making sense of it—culling through copious amounts of clinical and transactional information to determine relevance and gain insights to guide decisions and bring value to all departments and individuals touched by the supply chain on a regular basis.

Level V hospitals/health systems embrace their partners within and outside the organization as essential allies linked together through the flow of products and information. Contracting, purchasing, and receiving functions are largely centralized and automated throughout the enterprise. Operationally, the supply chain department has mostly mastered the *physical* flow of product and patient items—including their transportation, storage, and usage—and is on its way to mastering the *information* flow. Once accomplished, this will position the supply chain department to assume a more central role within the hospital/health system.

The principal opportunity for a Level V hospital/health system to move from "good to great" is expanding its reach—becoming *fully* centralized, working even *more* closely with clinicians and administrators, and striving to ensure that *all* decisions influenced or made by the supply chain are evidence-based and from a holistic CQO/patient-centered approach. With greater emphasis on cooperation, full use of metrics, and solid process-improvement methodologies, the supply chain department is on a trajectory to bring unquestioned value to the organization and to support the institution's efforts in fostering healthy communities in its catchment area.

Level V: Performance by Focus Area

Continuous Process Improvement (CPI)

Institutional CPI strategies include facilitating communication, information sharing, and prioritization to ensure implementation of supply chain business processes and existing technological solutions. At Level V, organizations apply CPI practices to supply chain functions and standardize CPI procedures and technologies across at least 75% of hospital/health system departments and/or service lines.

At this level, most tactics require substantial cooperation across departments and involve major collaboration among multiple disciplines. This is where the supply chain department can truly shine. Specifically, by owning the intersection of cost, quality, and outcomes, the department can lead change and firmly establish its value within the hospital/health system.

Contracting

At Level V, contracting services are largely centralized across the entire enterprise. Between 50% and 75% of the organization's spend is contracted. With this much spend accounted for, senior management is better positioned to control corporate contracting terms and practices and limit legal and financial liabilities. While a bit shy of best practice standards, Level V organizations are moving in the right direction in terms of contracting and cost, quality, and outcomes measures.

The hospital/health system works closely with its national and regional aggregation GPOs, as applicable, to leverage their buying power and services. The national GPO is utilized for 50%–75% of the organization's purchasing spend. All contracts are electronically activated, validated, and maintained; a streamlined electronic process allows for contract loading, notification of new products or price changes, and price synchronization with suppliers and distributors.

At Level V, some GPO contract categories are locally negotiated. The hospital/health system is making generally good use of its GPO membership, but it is not taking full advantage of the array of GPO products and services, including clinical support, benchmarking data, and reporting tools. Making better use of these services and tools could help the supply chain department synthesize cost data with quality and outcomes data, thereby approaching supply chain management from a more holistic CQO perspective.

The hospital/health system uses a competitive bidding process in its local contracting efforts. The process accounts for cost and quality measures but generally overlooks outcomes. Requiring locally negotiated contracts to include actual or projected reimbursement data in the bidding process will help the hospital/health system strengthen its performance in this area.

Data Management

Regardless of the supply management policies, processes, and technologies used by a hospital/health system, quality data are required. Detailed supply information and on-site supply data expertise can be hard to come by, making the IMF of paramount importance. Level V hospitals/health systems have a single item file that serves as the central repository for supply data and is updated at least quarterly. While this practice puts the hospital/health system leaps and bounds above many of its peers, implementing a formal process to ensure data integrity and updating the IMF daily (or as often as necessary) to ensure it is current would usher the institution into "top flight status" for data management from a CQO perspective.

Internal reports (by department, service line, and enterprise-wide) that reveal trends in practice and usage are created and used occasionally by decision makers in all aspects of supply chain management. Trend reports for internal *and* external comparisons (e.g., my hospital vs. peers) are generated and used periodically to make evidence-based decisions and influence practices related to contracting and purchasing.

Charges are captured in the CDM, and CDM maintenance occurs at least quarterly. The institution could boost revenue performance by prioritizing the CDM to ensure it encompasses *all* supply charges for *all* departments and is maintained daily or as often as necessary to ensure it is current.

Systems and/or processes exist to link the IMF to CDM, thereby providing the Level V hospital/health system with accurate item-level purchase and charge data comparisons.

Current IMF, CDM, and reporting data management practices place Level V hospitals/health systems in the upper range of the spectrum in the CQO framework.

Distribution

Supply chain integrity involves minimizing risks that arise anywhere along the supply chain—including distribution. Good distribution practices support sound business practices. Level V hospitals/health systems have a set distribution schedule that is posted, updated regularly, and adhered to in critical clinical and support areas. Supply distribution to departments and units outside of these two areas is not as reliable.

Shoring up distribution practices to incorporate a set distribution schedule that is observed enterprise-wide will build trust in the supply chain department and encourage clinicians and administrative staff to adhere to policies and procedures that meet their needs. Following a set distribution schedule is also essential for organizations seeking to meet the standards for the highest CQO level.

Education and Training

Formal supply chain instruction takes on an even greater role in the post-healthcare reform era. As supply chain departments embrace the CQO operational model, there will be greater collaboration with physicians and other clinical staff and coordination with other departments, so the importance of supply chain education and training will grow.

Level V hospitals/health systems view education and training as mission-critical and strive to ensure that staff has appropriate training, knowledge, experience, skills, and competence to perform its roles and responsibilities. As such, they have established formal clinical *and* non-clinical education and training programs for hospital/health system staff. Formal training programs are offered at least twice a year.

To take supply chain practices to the next level, supply chain–specific education and training should be fully integrated throughout the enterprise and take place on a routine, ongoing basis.

Internal Controls

Level V hospitals/health systems have established a process to identify, assess, and understand the critical areas in their supply chains. Formal supply chain–related internal controls have been developed and incorporated into all aspects of supply chain operations. Supply chain policies and procedures are integrated into the education and training program for clinical and non-clinical staff, are reviewed and updated at least annually, and are adhered to most of the time. A policy and procedure manual has been developed and is used by all departments and units throughout the organization.

The hospital/health system conducts internal audits sporadically and only on select supply chain processes. An internal audit plays a key role in the overall health of the organization by supporting senior management's efforts to improve and advance supply chain performance and excellence. To do so, internal auditors must regard the supply chain as an *integrated* process and evaluate supply chain performance universally (from a strategic perspective) as opposed to auditing supply chain functions and processes individually (from a tactical perspective). The audit process must also encompass procurement system audits as most of the transactions go through an automated system. Policies and procedures must be created not just for the supply chain department but across all departments involved in the procure-to-pay process.

Inventory Management

Level V hospitals/health systems employ sophisticated methods to track and manage inventory. Computerized point-of-use and enterprise asset management systems continuously record changes in both inventory quantity and inventory cost for most major inventory areas throughout the organization.

The hospital/health system uses a perpetual inventory system for the organization's storeroom, nursing units, and all other primary inventory locations such as operating rooms, radiology, the cath lab, etc. Real-time tracking reflects current inventory levels for each item in all locations; inventory is recorded each time inventory is touched or moved. Inventory is maintained routinely with scheduled manual inventory counts in the storeroom and nursing units; however, other major inventory locations are not maintained consistently.

PAR levels exist for all clinical areas. The numbers are reviewed quarterly, and performance is monitored directly by clinical operations' leadership. Level V organizations make partial use of automated dispensing systems, which offer a variety of benefits to the organization and staff and greatly support the organization's transition to a more holistic CQO approach. The automated dispensing systems provide nurses with near-total access to needed items in patient care areas, which decreases the delivery turnaround time of new items ordered. Increasing these systems' use from partial to full will ensure greater control of the charge capture of patient items and support security measures.

Cycle counting to verify inventory accuracy is performed regularly for all items in clinical departments and upon refill in automated dispensing systems. In all other (non-clinical) departments, cycle counting is executed only periodically.

Level V hospitals/health systems use an electronic charge-to-order system, which processes 75%–90% of all patient items. The charge-to-order system is particularly significant from a CQO perspective because the information it gathers aids the supply chain department in revenue capture and provides patient data that can be used in future clinical analyses and reimbursement scenarios. Best practices dictate that *at least* 90% of all patient items used enterprise-wide be on a charge-to-order system, so Level V organizations are performing well on this metric.

Policy setting, performance monitoring through sophisticated systems, and increased communication and compliance measures with clinical staff all contribute to dynamic and thorough inventory management practices, yet unvalued inventory still exists. In Level V hospitals/health systems, unvalued inventory represents more than 10% but less than 25% of inventory in any department or location.

The supply chain department uses a JIT strategy to reduce inventory and associated carrying costs. The focus is having "the right product, at the right place, at the right time." JIT is considered state-of-the-art in current inventory management systems. In Level V hospitals/health systems, the central storeroom houses and delivers emergency stock, and JIT is used in individual departments but not enterprise-wide.

Just-in-Time (JIT)
An inventory control system that controls material flow into assembly and manufacturing plants by coordinating demand and supply to the point where desired materials arrive just in time for use. An inventory reduction strategy, it feeds production lines with products delivered JIT. Developed by the auto industry, it refers to shipping goods in smaller, more frequent lots.

More than 16 active inventory turns in the hospital/health system occur annually, so inventory gets turned on a fairly regular basis. Although the hospital/health system uses a perpetual inventory system and JIT program, inactive inventory still represents up to 20% of total inventory value. Implementing the JIT program throughout the entire organization should help the supply chain department decrease its percentage of inactive inventory to low single digits.

Fewer than 200 stock-outs occur throughout the hospital/health system annually in Level V organizations, placing them in the upper range of the CQO spectrum. Increased monitoring and tighter inventory controls will help the organization reduce stock-outs and reach top-tier benchmarks—fewer than 100 stock-outs per year.

Purchasing

EDI is considered essential for supply chain departments wanting to build a successful, efficient, CQO-based purchasing program. At Level V, almost all of the medical, surgical, laboratory, and pharmacy items that the hospital/health system secures through its prime distributors are purchased using an EDI system. EDI is used for up to 50% of all other items purchased system-wide, and up to 75% of all purchase-line activity. EDI use accounts for half of the total spend of the organization.

Hospitals/health systems rated at Level V in purchasing could improve productivity and performance levels by making full use of the hospital's EDI system. EDI benefits include real-time transactional analysis, better forecasting, and lower inventory levels, all while reducing or eliminating human error.

To support the purchasing function, there is electronic three- to four-way price/quantity matching (contract→P.O.→receipt→invoice reconciliation) for all vendors and/or items. Three- to four-way price/quantity matching is used for up to 75% of all purchase lines and 50% of the organization's total spend.

As a result of established processes and system automation, purchasing staff can focus on value-added activities rather than transactional tasks.

Receiving

A centralized receiving process is in place for both stock and non-stock purchases in Level V hospitals/health systems. All deliveries are received at the loading dock and loaded into the MMIS via handheld devices. Many stock items received from the distributor are prepackaged for delivery to storeroom inventory locations; however, the supply chain does not follow a regular timetable for sending items to storerooms. To improve supply chain performance in this area and move to Level VI, the organization should concentrate on increasing the number of prepackaged items and adhering to a set schedule for sending products to storerooms.

At least 75% of all hospital/health system departments and service lines adhere to the organization's non-stock receiving policies and procedures.

Reimbursement

Most Level V hospitals/health systems recognize the value that accompanies supply chain improvement, and, as a result, invest significantly in the technology, staff, and equipment to achieve such ends. Metrics that document supply chain performance and track changes over time are the department's way of showing a return on that investment.

To be truly effective, supply chain measurement must link operational performance to the hospital/health system's strategy and create a means by which to identify the issues, challenges, and obstacles that could keep the organization from achieving its long-term strategic goals.

Organizations operating at Level V continuously capture and track supply cost and revenue metrics as well as develop dashboards and sophisticated reports that show trends and supply performance measures other than traditional cost and performance variances. Those analytics are used periodically (but not routinely) to support decision making at the unit, department, or administration level. By leading from a CQO-grounded perspective, the supply chain department can educate hospital/health system staff, improve communications, and ensure that advanced analytical capabilities are available, understood, and used routinely to support enterprise-wide decision making.

Requisitioning

For Level V hospitals/health systems, an electronic requisitioning system is used by at least 75% of all departments and service lines. This provides a positive requisitioning experience for staff, which in turn encourages all employees in the hospital/health system to drive purchases through a paperless process and allows the supply chain department to capture valuable data about enterprise-wide purchasing. Electronic requisitioning accounts for up to 50% of all purchase lines and 40% of the total spend purchased organization-wide.

The remaining 25% of requests for goods and services are generated manually, making it more difficult to regulate and track. While this is a strong performance depicting an organization headed in the right direction, tightening up policies and practices in e-procurement will enable the supply chain department to operate more consistently from the CQO perspective, and bring greater value to the departments and units with which it is integrally related.

Value Analysis

Value analysis programs in Level V hospitals/health systems reflect an inter-disciplinary culture that supports the integration of supply chain and cost reduction within clinical operations. Collaboration is more than a buzzword in these institutions—it is part of the very fabric that weaves individual departmental strategies with the organization's overall strategy and helps the hospital/health system achieve successful financial and clinical outcomes.

A physician-led Value Analysis Steering Committee directs the value analysis program. Physician team members regularly rotate on and off the committee to allow all physician leaders an opportunity to contribute to the value analysis process and to allow supply chain leaders an opportunity to engage and involve the clinical community in the CQO approach to product and technology selection.

The supply chain is almost fully integrated with clinical operations, working closely with clinicians and focusing on high-volume procedures and service lines to drive down costs, increase patient safety, and foster positive clinical outcomes. At Level V, the supply chain department is recognized for the unique and strategic role it plays in coordinating across hospital/health system clinical and administrative departments to maximize efficiency and value as well as evaluate procedure-specific revenues and expenses to achieve financial targets.

Patient-Centered Care
The Institute of Medicine defines patient-centered care as: Health care that establishes a partnership among practitioners, patients, and their families (when appropriate) to ensure that decisions respect patients' wants, needs, and preferences and that patients have the education and support they need to make decisions and participate in their own care.

Clinical and non-clinical products, services, and technologies are introduced into the hospital/health system after a thorough vetting by an interdepartmental committee comprising key stakeholders (e.g., finance, supply chain, performance improvement, clinical). Multidisciplinary teams evaluate 50%–75% of new products and services prior to purchase.

The hospital/health system's approach to value analysis demonstrates that CQO has become an integral part of the organization. There is an enterprise-wide continuous process of establishing cost-, quality- and outcomes-driven initiatives. Interdepartmental data-sharing and evidence-based practices are common, and the organization is clearly focused on patient-centered care.

LEVEL VI

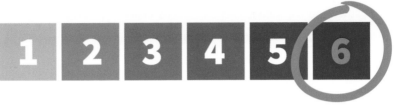

Overall Composite Score

Hospitals/health systems that achieve an overall score of Level VI on the Self-Assessment represent the top tier of supply chain management performance. In these institutions, the supply chain is no longer viewed as just another department or division; rather, it is seen as a complex set of functions that are woven into the very fabric of the organization and thus are integral to the institution's success and fundamental to the achievement of CQO goals. Supply chain executives are recognized for their vision, efficiency, and resourcefulness by clinicians and administrators across the organization.

Level VI hospitals/health systems are characterized by their patient-centered approach with a significant focus on the patients and their experience, which translates into all aspects of supply chain management from planning and purchasing to inventory, logistics, and distribution. This is particularly evident in their use of tools and technology to acquire, analyze, and use data, as well as in their use of tools and technology to share that intelligence with relevant parties to inform purchasing decisions.

The strategies and methodologies employed to achieve this level of operation are decidedly collaborative, with supply chain department staff represented on and working closely with internal teams and departments throughout the organization. The supply chain department also fosters and enjoys strong relationships with external companies and organizations, working with suppliers to eliminate bottlenecks and avoid overstock, practicing strategic sourcing and implementing JIT techniques to streamline operations and optimize the workings of the entire supply chain.

Like their clinical counterparts, evolved supply chain departments are driven by data and practice their own version of evidence-based healthcare. They gather and use data from wide and diverse resources, looking for trends, waste, and inefficiencies in the supply chain. Data drive innovation, spark cooperation, and lie at the core of all strategic decision making. Because the supply chain department captures, analyzes, and uses valid and reliable data, it acts authoritatively, advises and influences opinions, and leads from a position solidly grounded in the CQO approach.

At this highly evolved level of supply chain management, processes are almost entirely automated and integrated across the organization. All focus areas—from contracting to purchasing to receiving to inventory management—use leading-edge technologies to implement procedures and collect, manage, and track data. Data are linked and shared between systems to inform decision making, expedite delivery of goods and services, and otherwise advance excellence across the supply chain.

A "culture of excellence" further defines Level VI organizations. A firm commitment to education and CPI exists, which is reflected in the ethos of the supply chain department and is exhibited by everyone on the supply chain team. Ongoing education, training, and mentoring are supported and encouraged, formally and informally. The culture of excellence is also evident in the supply chain department's internal controls. Standardized processes, procedures, and technologies are implemented, used enterprise-wide, and routinely evaluated and updated.

Level VI: Performance by Focus Area

Continuous Process Improvement (CPI)

At Level VI, the organization uses a top-notch suite of tools and concepts to drive supply chain operational process excellence across the entire enterprise. CPI processes, procedures, and technology are standardized and used by at least 90% of hospital/health system departments and service lines. Through CPI, the supply chain department delivers optimized, value-added benefits for patients, employees, and the institution as a whole. The hospital/health system, particularly the supply chain department, encourages and supports a culture of innovation grounded in CQO to improve operational efficiencies. Supply chain staff is committed to the concept of CPI and actively participates in strategic discussions to develop, enhance, and refine processes in their unit.

CPI processes and procedures are continuously evaluated to ensure waste is eliminated and the focus remains on streamlining efficiencies throughout the hospital/health system's entire supply chain.

Contracting

At Level VI, contracting services operate like a well-oiled machine. Contracting is centralized across the entire enterprise to increase efficiency, streamline spend, reduce duplication of common activities across projects and departments, and allow senior management to establish better control of institutional contracting terms and practices. For hospitals/health systems operating at Level VI, more than 75% of the organization's purchasing spend is contracted.

The hospital/health system's national GPO is used for more than 75% of its spend. Contracting services are automated to expedite purchasing and reduce human error. All contracts are electronically activated, validated, and maintained.

Some GPO contract categories are locally negotiated and, in such instances, contracted suppliers are required to report spend to the GPO. Local contracts are developed using a competitive bidding process that shares terms, conditions, and bid evaluation criteria in an open and transparent manner with potential bidders. A well-developed contracting program also makes extensive use of the broad array of services available through its GPO (e.g., networking, benchmarking, and education).

Contracting is conducted from a patient-centered perspective so that, in addition to cost considerations, the quality of the goods and services and evidence-based clinical outcomes are factored into the procurement process.

Data Management

Data management represents the foremost opportunity for hospitals/health systems to recover revenue and maximize reimbursement. Organizations distinguish themselves at Level VI through meticulous use of the IMF and CDM as well as through sophisticated use of reports.

There is one item file that is updated daily (or as often as is necessary) to ensure all records are current and user-defined information about each item is maintained. A formal process has been implemented to certify data integrity, and third party IMF maintenance is used to validate all necessary information. Additionally, detailed product information and business rules enhance data for downstream systems and reporting. A dedicated data management team controls all information added to the IMF. Similarly, only one CDM exists, and it is maintained daily. Hospitals/health systems typically use an automated CDM tool that standardizes pricing and descriptions for line items and monitors for regulatory compliance; if there is no automated tool, manual updates are systematically performed pursuant to established policies and procedures. Interfaces that support data flow across systems are also established to create standardized information stemming from the supply chain data source.

Reports that show trends and variances are used routinely throughout the hospital/health system to make evidence-based decisions regarding contracting, purchasing, and policies associated with item use.

Distribution

In Level VI hospitals/health systems, distribution is available to support the needs of clinicians, special units, and all departments twenty-four hours a day, seven days a week. Medical/surgical supplies are distributed according to a set schedule that is current and adhered to throughout the institution. The distribution department plays an integral role in CQO by providing patient care–related items on a timely basis across the organization.

Education and Training

Ongoing education and training is vital in healthcare, where technology changes rapidly and research that improves quality and efficiency emerges regularly. Formal clinical and non-clinical supply chain–related education and training is a top priority for Level VI hospitals/health systems. A culture of excellence extends to every aspect of supply chain management, and the supply chain department's dedication to achieving and maintaining state-of-the-art supply chain operations is reflected in its education program and commitment to developing its professionals to their maximum potential.

General classes and specialized training are offered on an ongoing basis. Training is integrated throughout the enterprise and involves the participation of all key internal and external stakeholders.

Internal Controls

Level VI organizations maintain a set of vetted and well-documented internal controls that are integral components of the internal audit plan. Supply chain internal controls encourage efficiency and compliance with laws, codes and regulations, and hospital/health system policies. Additionally, they are designed to expose and eliminate waste, fraud, and abuse. These policies and procedures are kept current and are consistently adhered to enterprise-wide. Supply chain department directors and managers are responsible for estab-lishing and maintaining internal controls within their units. All supply chain personnel are responsible for *executing* the internal controls established by their units. Individuals have been educated and trained on their responsibilities as they relate to the overall policies and procedures for the department, and ongoing education is encouraged.

Inventory Management

While many factors affect the management of inventory, the inventory management systems of Level VI hospitals/health systems are primarily distinguished by their accounting method, delivery system, use of automation, the number of active inventory turns, and the percentage of unvalued inventory.

Perpetual inventory exists and is maintained routinely for all inventory locations throughout the hospital/health system. All inventory is accounted for in near real time through computerized point-of-sale and enterprise-wide asset management systems to provide a detailed assessment of changes in inventory and to allow real-time reporting of the amount of inventory in stock.

At Level VI, *all* clinical areas account for inventory with PAR levels and employ full use of automated dispensing systems to ensure all necessary products and patient items are in stock and available as needed. PAR levels are reviewed monthly by clinical operations leadership, and any relevant information or observations are shared with supply chain management. Supply chain reporting is used to recommend PAR level updates and, as possible, occurs in real time. Cycle counts are performed on a regularly scheduled basis in all clinical and non-clinical departments, and also occur upon refill of automated dispensing systems.

Patient charges can significantly affect patient satisfaction scores, one of several metrics to define CQO. In sophisticated supply chains, more than 90% of patient items are processed via a charge-to-order system.

In Level VI hospitals/health systems, there is *no* unvalued inventory. All locations and departments maintain a current and accurate accounting of their inventory so that the organization always knows its exact value. Inactive inventory represents 10% or less of the total value of inventory. Stock integrity is verified through multiple active inventory turns; more than 20 inventory turns are performed annually in the hospital or in each facility within a health system.

"Just in Case" is nonexistent; JIT is used throughout the hospital/health system. Managers can accurately forecast demand and keep inventory to a minimum. A JIT system is established enterprise-wide, assuring that supplies are received only as they are needed, thereby significantly reducing inventory costs. The hospital/health system storeroom houses and delivers emergency stock. This level of operation is further defined by the fact that fewer than 100 stock-outs occur in the institution annually.

Purchasing

Highly developed supply chain purchasing programs are distinguished by the percentage of purchases made through an EDI system. At Level VI, EDI is established throughout the organization and used for at least 75% of all items purchased. EDI also represents at least 85% of all purchase lines and 70% of the total spend purchased.

Purchases processed electronically match the invoice information with supporting documentation. There is at least a "three-way match" and optimally a "five-way match" of the price and quantity of goods or services purchased. Specifically, the system matches: 1) the invoice to 2) the P.O. and 3) the packing slip or equivalent (e.g., receipt slip, bill of lading). More evolved organizations reflect a full five-way match, adding contract compliance and reimbursement reconciliation to the process. This safeguards against payments being made out of compliance (resulting in overpayments) and ensures adherence with all discounts and special terms.

Receiving

Hospitals/health systems operating at Level VI have a well-established, highly automated receiving operation. Receiving policy and procedures are thoroughly documented for clarity and instructional purposes. The receiving process is regulated by an online scheduling system to manage and streamline deliveries.

For stock purchases, without exception, all deliveries to the institution are received at the loading dock. Pallets and JIT inventories are scanned upon delivery via handheld technology and the data are uploaded into the MMIS. The majority of all stock items are received at the facility through a coordinated distributor and are prepackaged for immediate delivery to storeroom inventory locations.

Global Location Number (GLN)
The GS1 Identification Key used for any location (physical, operational, or legal) that needs to be identified for use in the supply chain. The GLN is a globally unique number that can be used to access master data about a location.

Receiving procedures for non-stock purchases are dictated by a centralized process to which all departments and service lines adhere. When the Global Location Number® system is fully implemented by suppliers and other key supply chain participants, hospitals/health systems operating at Level VI will fully use this system.

Reimbursement

At this most advanced level, the supply chain department optimizes reimbursement by using state-of-the art data. Metrics that reflect supply cost, the quality of goods and services, patient satisfaction and experience, and outcomes are routinely captured, tracked, and used to support purchasing decisions throughout the organization.

The supply chain department gathers and uses data from key sources throughout the organization (MMIS, finance, risk management, environmental services, support services, value analysis teams, etc.) along with useful external data (e.g., Truven, AHRQ) to arm supply chain executives and other decision makers with the information needed to understand how purchasing decisions, supply usage, and supply chain operations affect reimbursement.

Requisitioning

The requisitioning process in Level VI organizations is almost entirely automated. In these hospitals/health systems, at least 90% of the organization's departments or service lines use an online/electronic system to request purchases. The requisition is submitted and routed electronically for necessary departmental approvals, at which time it is converted to a purchase order. The electronic requisitions also actively monitor requestor selections and prompt the user to select contracted items, which have been evaluated using CQO methodology. The automated system gives the reviewer the ability to check parameters of the requisition regarding inventory levels and financial controls. At this level, the electronic requisitioning system represents *at least* 75% of all purchase lines and 65% of the total spend purchased.

Value Analysis

Level VI hospitals/health systems have value analysis programs grounded in the CQO model. Many departments are involved in and contribute at various levels to the value analysis process—physicians, other clinicians, information technology, finance, risk management—but the supply chain *owns* the intersection of cost, quality, and outcomes, and manages the process from this intersection. Physicians, in particular, play a significant role in value analysis at this level, as they provide executive oversight to all of the organization's value analysis teams and lead the Value Analysis Steering Committee. While physicians provide direction to the committees and the decision-making process, they seek out and solicit input and participation from all key stakeholders including finance, supply chain, performance improvement, risk management, environmental services, sustainability coordinators, caregivers, etc. The process is driven with a constant focus on clinical outcomes and value.

There is a two-tiered process for the introduction and adoption of new clinical and non-clinical products, services, and technologies. At this advanced level, an interdepartmental committee comprising stakeholders integral to the relevant service line evaluates more than 75% of new products and services. If the committee selects a product or service, it is vetted and tested for clinical effectiveness by a technology committee before being introduced for widespread use throughout the hospital/health system.

CQO is symbolic of the philosophy of the organization. The Value Analysis Steering Committee and value analysis teams reflect all of the key stakeholders across the organization. They employ processes and safeguards that ensure all initiatives are evidence-based and continuously reviewed from a CQO perspective. The focus is patient centered, and reimbursement rates, patient satisfaction scores, and outcomes data are fully integrated in the decision-making process.

Achieving Level VI

Improving Supply Chain Performance … One Step at a Time

Results from the Self-Assessment provide valuable insight into the strengths and weaknesses of the supply chain at the individual focus–area level. These results should form the basis of an actionable supply chain performance improvement and implementation plan. Ideally, resources permitting, all focus areas that score below a Level VI should be tackled simultaneously; however, this isn't likely to be feasible for most organizations, so priorities should be established based on the organization's strategic objectives.

The following describes the individual focus areas and the characteristics that differentiate levels within each area. This information is intended to guide efforts to attain Level VI both within each focus area as well as overall.

Continuous Process Improvement (CPI)

CPI: Level VI

CPI processes, procedures, and technology are standardized across at least 90% of hospital departments and/or service lines and are continuously evaluated to eliminate waste and improve efficiency.

CPI is the "ongoing effort to improve products, services, or processes. These efforts can seek 'incremental' improvement over time or 'breakthrough' improvement all at once."[29] The origins of CPI can be traced to the Japanese strategy known as *kaizen* or "good change." *Kaizen* was originally used by Japanese businesses after WWII, particularly in the manufacturing industry by Toyota. While the manufacturers have used these methods successfully for many years, the concept has more recently been adopted and implemented in other industries including healthcare.[30] Drawing from the *kaizen* playbook,[31] CPI seeks to reduce waste and increase value for customers through continuous improvements.

---

[29] "Continuous Improvement," *American Society for Quality*, accessed August 5, 2014, http://asq.org/learn-about-quality/continuous-improvement/overview/overview.html.

[30] J. Weed, "Factory Efficiency Comes to the Hospital," *New York Times*, July 10, 2010, http://www.nytimes.com/2010/07/11/business/11seattle.html?_r=0.

[31] M. Imai, *Kaizen: The Key to Japan's Competitive Success* (New York: McGraw-Hill/Irwin, 1986).

Hospitals and other healthcare organizations use CPI to improve everyday processes in clinical and administrative departments to foster greater operational efficiency. This involves identifying problems that obstruct workflow processes, formulating and implementing process improvement solutions, and evaluating the impact of the improvements. CPI, as reflected in its name, is a continuous process; thus, it should be an inherent element of each and every clinical and administrative unit. Done well, CPI efforts will lead to improved efficiency, reduced costs, and improvements in quality of care.[32,33,34]

Under the CQO framework, Level I organizations are characterized by having no CPI processes, procedures, or technology in place, while the opposite end of the spectrum (Level VI) is characterized by employing CPI virtually enterprise-wide. The intervening levels reflect the gradual adoption and dissemination of CPI strategies across the organization. So, for example, an organization with no CPI processes, procedures, or technology in place (Level I) can move to Level II simply by instituting *some* CPI processes, procedures, and technology in one or more departments and/or service lines, even if these are variable. The *standardization* of CPI processes, procedures, and technologies in some departments and/or service lines is a significant step and earns an organization a Level III ranking. The remaining three performance levels are distinguished by the extent to which the now standardized CPI processes, procedures, and technology are implemented throughout the organization. Specifically, CPI processes, procedures, and technology are standardized across at least 50% of departments and/or service lines in Level IV organizations, at least 75% of departments and/or service lines in Level V organizations, and 90% of departments and/or service lines in Level VI organizations. Level V and VI organizations are further distinguished by the addition of CPI *evaluation* activities conducted

---

[32] S. Rodak, "What Continuous Improvement Looks Like in a Hospital OR: Lean at ThedaCare," *Becker's Hospital Review*, September 12, 2011, http://www.beckershospitalreview.com/or-efficiencies/what-continuous-improvement-looks-like-in-a-hospital-or-lean-at-thedacare.html.

[33] I. Andrabi, "A Culture of Continuous Improvement Is Necessary for Success Under Value-Based Care," *Becker's Hospital Review*, February 23, 2012, http://www.beckershospitalreview.com/hospital-management-administration/a-culture-of-continuous-improvement-is-necessary-for-success-under-value-based-care.html .

[34] The MITRE Institute, *MITRE Systems Engineering (SE) Competency Model, Version 1, September 1, 2007* (Mitre Corporation: 2010), http://www.mitre.org/sites/default/files/publications/10_0678_presentation.pdf.

on a periodic basis (Level V) and on a continuous basis with emphasis on eliminating waste and improving efficiency (Level VI).

Contracting

Contracting is a key element of the CQO framework because effective contracting yields the best possible prices for supplies, products, and services, which, in turn, contribute to achieving the objective of delivering the highest quality care at the lowest possible cost. Under the CQO framework, the Contracting focus area is measured by three attributes: centralized, enterprise-wide contracting control and purchasing; group purchasing organization (GPO) contracting; and local contracting.

In Level I organizations, there is no centralized contracting process; the organization is not affiliated with a formal GPO, and local contracts, as a general rule, are not competitively bid or developed with much (if any) cost consideration.

Contracting Control & Purchasing: Level VI

More than 75% of spend is contracted, and contracting is centralized across the enterprise.

With respect to **contracting control and purchasing**, the CQO framework rests on the assumption that this function is centralized because centralization appears 1) to be the best way to guarantee rigor and account-ability in purchasing practices enterprise-wide, and 2) to ensure the best product quality and pricing is secured across the organization. Centralization can result in excessive bureaucracy and lack of responsiveness, which can be avoided by instituting and adhering to appropriate policies and procedures, thereby ensuring the benefits of centralization outweigh the risks. At Level II, there is a centralized contracting process, but individuals or individual departments negotiate their own contracts with vendors of their choosing. Thereafter, the CQO performance levels in the contracting arena reflect the successive amounts of supply spend that are contracted (i.e., less than 25% of spend is contracted in a Level III organization, 25% to less than 50% in a

Level IV organization, 50%–75% in a Level V organization, and more than 75% in a Level VI organization) coupled with the extent to which contracting is centralized across the organization (i.e., contracting is partially centralized in a Level III organization, moving toward full centralization in a Level IV organization, largely centralized in a Level V organization, and fully centralized in a Level VI organization).

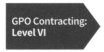

The primary GPO is utilized for more than 75% of spend; contracts are electronically activated, validated, and maintained; some GPO contract categories are locally negotiated with mandatory supplier GPO reporting; and there is broad use of additional GPO services.

On the **GPO contracting** front, studies have shown that GPOs provide significant value to participating healthcare organizations.[35] Accordingly, a key benchmark in the CQO framework is the extent to which an organization purchases products and services through GPO contracts and uses the broad array of other services offered by GPOs including, for example, tools and technology that support online management of contracts and pricing, benchmarking against peer organizations, and quality and outcomes analytics. Thus, a Level II organization is characterized by affiliations with one or more GPOs, although purchases made through GPO contracts are done on a selective case-by-case basis. In contrast, a Level VI organization uses its primary GPO for more than 75% of spend; contracts are electronically activated, validated, and maintained; and there is broad use of additional GPO services. Successive improvements are measured by increasing the amount an organization spends through GPO contracts and greater use of GPO services. Level III organizations are affiliated with one or more GPOs, but less than 50% of spend is through GPO contracts. Level IV organizations use a primary or secondary GPO for contract pricing and electronic activation for at least

---

[35] See, for example, *The Role of Group Purchasing Organizations in the US Health Care System*, a report prepared by Muse & Associates for HIGPA (Washington, DC, March, 2000), https://www.novationco.com/media/industryinfo/MuseStudy.pdf; and E. S. Schneller, *The Value of Group Purchasing—2009: Meeting the Needs for Strategic Savings* (Healthcare Sector Advances, supported by data from Mathematica Research, April 2009), https://www.novationco.com/media/industryinfo/value_of_gpo_2009.pdf.

50% of product purchases, and there is partial use of other GPO services. Level V organizations use their primary GPO for 50%–75% of spend; contracts are electronically activated, validated, and maintained; and there is material use of additional GPO services.

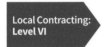

Local contracts are developed for all projects using a competitive bidding process and focus on cost, quality, and outcomes.

Finally, with respect to **local contracting**, Level II organizations develop local contracts using a competitive bidding process sporadically and with some consideration for costs. At Level III, local contracts are developed for major projects using a competitive bidding process but only focus on cost. At Level IV, virtually all local contracts are competitively bid but still focus only on cost. At Level V, local contracts are competitively bid (at least for all major projects) and focus on both cost and quality. Lastly, Level VI performance is characterized by using a competitive bidding process in all instances, focusing on cost, quality, and outcomes.

Data Management

The importance of data and data management in supply chain operations cannot be overstated. Successful supply chain operations—within and across focus areas and for the supply chain as a whole—hinge on the availability and use of accurate and timely data. While data and data management permeate all elements of the supply chain, the CQO framework focuses on three specific areas—**item master file (IMF)**, reporting, and charge capture—for purposes of measuring performance in data management.

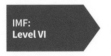

There is a single item file that is updated daily or as often as necessary to ensure that it is current. A formal process is in place to ensure data integrity.

An item master file is a live computerized record of the individual items an organization uses. It captures essential and comprehensive information about each item, including (as applicable) manufacturer, vendor, item number, product number, catalog number, description, pricing, unit of measure, ABC code, and so forth. At its core, the IMF standardizes information for requisitioning, purchasing, analytics, and enterprise-wide downstream systems and reporting. Level I organizations have no IMF. In Level II organizations, there are individual item files, but these files are not maintained. In Level III organizations, there are multiple item files, but they are individually managed and updated less than quarterly. Level IV organizations have multiple item files that are updated and transitioned into one consolidated IMF, but IMF maintenance is sporadic. At Level V, there is a single IMF, which is updated at least quarterly. Finally, at Level VI, there is a single IMF that is updated daily or as often as necessary to ensure it is current, and there is a formal process in place to ensure data integrity.

Reporting: Level VI

Trend reports for internal and external comparisons (e.g., my hospital vs. peers) are used routinely.

On the **reporting** front, there are no reports generated or available in Level I organizations. At Level II, basic transactional reports are available, and at Level III, static "point-in-time" reports are generated. Level IV institutions generate trend reports (by department, service line, and enterprise), but they are used only periodically. At Level V, trend reports for internal and external comparisons (e.g., my hospital vs. peers) are generated, but again, they are used only periodically. At Level VI, internal and external trend reports are generated and used routinely.

Charge Capture: Level VI

A CDM encompasses all supply charges for all departments and is maintained daily or as often as necessary to ensure it is current.

Finally, with respect to **charge capture**, there is little to no charge capture in Level I organizations. At Level II, supply charges are captured, but are not tracked with an accurate charge description master (CDM), the master price list of patient charges for supplies, devices, medications, services, procedures, etc. At Level III, there is a CDM, but maintenance is minimal. Likewise, at Level IV, a CDM is in place, and maintenance occurs more frequently but still less than quarterly. Finally, a CDM is in place and maintenance occurs at least quarterly at Level V and as often as necessary to ensure it is current at Level VI.

Distribution

Distribution Schedule: Level VI

There is a set supply distribution schedule that is up-to-date and adhered to enterprise-wide.

The distribution department is responsible for the ongoing delivery of medical/surgical supplies; patient care equipment (e.g., beds, isolation carts, and liquid oxygen and nitrogen); and other patient supplies as well as the rotation and replenishment of exchange carts, case carts, etc. Distribution, closely tied to receiving and inventory management, is essential for ensuring hospitals/health systems operate with maximum efficiency, thereby minimizing or eliminating unnecessary costs associated with discharge or operating room delays, etc. In the CQO framework, "distribution schedule" is the key attribute, where performance ranges from no set supply distribution schedule (Level I) to a set supply distribution schedule that is up-to-date and adhered to enterprise-wide (Level VI). Levels in between reflect

- the maturing of the distribution process (e.g., at Level II, there is a set supply distribution schedule, but it is not adhered to and/or is frequently out-of-date, and at Level III, there is a set supply distribution schedule, but it is adhered to and/or updated only sporadically); and
- an enterprise rollout strategy (e.g., at Level IV, a set supply distribution schedule is updated regularly but adhered to only for critical clinical areas, while at Level V, a set supply distribution schedule is updated regularly and adhered to for critical clinical and support areas).

Educating and Training

Supply Chain
Education:
Level VI

Formal clinical and non-clinical supply chain-related education and training is fully integrated throughout the enterprise and takes place on a routine, ongoing basis.

Achieving the objectives of CQO hinges to a significant extent on educating and training clinicians and administrators in supply chain operations and related matters. Specifically, they need to have an in-depth understanding about the individual components of the supply chain; how each component operates; how the individual components are interconnected and interdependent; the positive clinical and financial consequences associated with a smoothly operating supply chain; and the ripple effects, disruptions, and costly consequences associated with the breakdown of any individual supply chain component. Moreover, clinicians in particular must be very knowledgeable about the products they use (e.g., cost, complications, and outcomes); quality indicators and measures; product-specific reimbursement policies (e.g., implantable devices); and overall payment policies (e.g., bundled payments and risk-sharing arrangements). Ideally, supply chain–related education and training, as described herein, should be formalized, ongoing, and targeted to all clinical and administrative staff.

On the CQO spectrum, education ranges from no formal clinical or non-clinical supply chain–related education and training (Level I) to formal clinical and non-clinical supply chain–related education where it is fully integrated throughout the enterprise and takes place on a routine, ongoing basis (Level VI). Movement from Level I to Level II is achieved simply by providing formal supply chain–related education and training during new-hire orientation. Subsequent levels are reached by providing formal clinical *or* non-clinical supply chain–related education and training at least once a year (Level III), clinical *and* non-clinical supply chain–related education at least once a year (Level IV), and clinical and non-clinical supply chain–related education at least twice a year (Level V).

Internal Controls

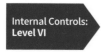

Formal supply chain-related internal controls, policies, and procedures are an integral component of the internal audit plan; these are always up-to-date and are consistently adhered to enterprise-wide.

Internal controls for supply chain–related activities are essential for ensuring the proper functioning of the supply chain on an ongoing basis. Hospitals/health systems typically have at least basic supply chain–related internal controls in place such as a method for recording supply deliveries and matching a purchase order with a receipt and an invoice. As organizations evolve within the CQO framework, internal controls tying explicitly to cost, quality, and outcomes must be instituted. Consequently, policies and procedures pertaining to all key elements of the supply chain (e.g., purchasing, requisitioning, data capture, etc.) should be written, implemented, monitored for adherence, reviewed and updated routinely, and audited regularly.

- Level I organizations are characterized by having no formal supply chain–related internal controls, policies, and procedures.
- Level II organizations have such policies and procedures, but there is no process in place to ensure they are current.
- Level III organizations have formal policies and procedures, but they are neither maintained in a timely manner nor enforced.
- Level IV organizations have formal policies and procedures that are reviewed and updated at least annually, but they are not adhered to consistently and are audited infrequently (less than every three years).
- Level V organizations have formal policies and procedures that are reviewed and updated at least annually and adhered to most of the time, and internal audits are conducted occasionally on selected processes.
- Level VI organizations have formal policies and procedures in place that are always up-to-date and consistently adhered to enterprise-wide. Moreover, the review of these policies and procedures is baked into the organization's internal audit plan.

Inventory Management

In the CQO framework, inventory management plays a fundamental role in controlling costs and achieving optimal operational efficiency. Inventory management is measured by eight attributes: charge-to-order system, cycle counting, inventory delivery system, inventory turns, PAR levels, perpetual inventory, stock-outs, and unvalued inventory. The following describes the organizational performance characteristics for these attributes.

Charge-to-Order System: Level VI

At least 90% of patient items are processed via a charge-to-order system.

There is no **charge-to-order** system in Level I organizations, and at Level II, charge-to-order is a manual process. Thereafter, charge-to-order is technology based with increasing amounts of patient items processed using charge-to-order software. Thus, the percentage of patient items processed via a charge-to-order system is 50% or fewer at Level III, more than 50% but less than 75% at Level IV, more than 75% but less than 90% at Level V, and at least 90% at Level VI.

Cycle Counting: Level VI

Cycle counting is performed in all departments regularly for all items in all clinical and non-clinical areas and upon refill in automated dispensing systems.

Cycle counting is a process or system for counting subsets of the total inventory on a regular basis throughout the year instead of the traditional once-a-year full inventory count.[36]

- In Level I organizations, no cycle counting is performed.
- At Level II, cycle counting is performed sporadically, but is not based on ABC analysis (the process of grouping items into three categories in order of their estimated importance, where "A" items are very important, "B" items are important, and "C" items are marginally important).[37]

---

[36] D. Piasecki, "Cycle Counting and Physical Inventories," InventoryOps.Com, accessed August 7, 2014, http://www.inventoryops.com/cycle_counting_and_physical_inventories.htm.

[37] "ABC Analysis," BusinessDictionary.com, accessed August 7, 2014, http://www.businessdictionary.com/definition/ABC-analysis.html#ixzz39ioPAXRo.

- Level III organizations perform cycle counting sporadically and/or in some major department areas, but it is still not based on ABC analysis.
- At Level IV, cycle counting takes place in major department areas regularly and is based on ABC analysis.
- At Level V, cycle counting is performed regularly for all clinical department items, periodically for non-clinical department items, and upon refill in automated dispensing systems.
- Finally, at Level VI, cycle counting occurs in all clinical and non-clinical areas regularly and upon refill in automated dispensing systems.

Inventory Delivery Systems: Level VI

The storeroom houses and delivers emergency stock, and a JIT program is in place and used enterprise-wide.

There are no formal **inventory delivery systems** in Level I organizations, except perhaps for emergency items. Level II organizations are characterized by high levels of inventory and some expired items in the storeroom, but the storeroom stocks some departments. At Level III, there are controlled levels of inventory in the storeroom, few to no expired items, and the storeroom stocks all hospital departments. At Levels IV, V, and VI, the storeroom houses and delivers emergency stock. In addition, individual departments in Level IV organizations are stocked using a LUM program; some departments are stocked using a JIT program at Level V; and at Level VI, a JIT program is in place and used enterprise-wide.

Inventory Turns: Level VI

There are more than 20 active inventory turns in the hospital annually; inactive inventory represents up to 10% of total inventory value.

The number of **annual inventory turns** performed by an organization and the amount of inactive inventory differentiates organizations across the performance levels. The following are examples:

- There are **0 to 4** active inventory turns, and inactive inventory exceeds 50% of total inventory value in Level I organizations.

- In Level II organizations, there are **5 to 8** annual active inventory turns, and inactive inventory represents up to 50% of total inventory value.
- Level III organizations have **9 to 12** active inventory turns annually, and inactive inventory represents up to 40% of total inventory value.
- At Level IV, there are **more than 12** annual active inventory turns, and inactive inventory represents up to 30% of total inventory value.
- At Level V, there are **more than 16** active inventory turns annually, and inactive inventory represents up to 20% of total inventory value.
- Finally, at the top level (Level VI), there are **more than 20** annual active inventory turns, and inactive inventory represents no more than 10% of total inventory value.

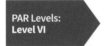
PAR Levels: Level VI

PAR levels exist for all clinical areas. They are reviewed monthly with performance monitored by clinical operations leadership, and they employ full use of automated dispensing systems.

Periodic automatic replacement or periodic automatic replenishment (PAR) provides for item restocking when inventories fall below predefined levels. In Level I institutions, there are no established PARs. At Level II, there are established PAR levels for major clinical areas, but the PARs are reviewed sporadically. Thereafter, there are PARs for all clinical areas, but the performance level is determined by the frequency of their review and other factors such as the degree of clinical leadership involvement in monitoring PARs and the use of automated dispensing systems. Thus, at Level III, PAR levels exist for *all* clinical areas, but are still reviewed only sporadically. At Level IV, PAR levels are reviewed at least annually, and performance is reported to clinical operations leadership. At Level V, PAR levels are reviewed quarterly, performance is monitored by clinical operations leadership, and the organization makes partial use of automated dispensing systems. Finally, at Level VI, PAR levels are reviewed monthly, performance is monitored by clinical operations leadership, and automated dispensing systems are fully employed.

| Perpetual Inventory: Level VI | *Perpetual inventory exists and is routinely maintained for all inventory locations.* |

Perpetual inventory refers to a computerized inventory management system that supports inventory management in near real time. At Level I, there is no perpetual inventory, and at Level II, inventory levels are maintained manually. At Level III, there is perpetual inventory in the organization's storeroom. At the remaining levels, perpetual inventory is expanded throughout the organization. So, perpetual inventory exists for the storeroom and nursing units at Level IV, but only the storeroom is maintained regularly. At Level V, perpetual inventory is in place for the storeroom, nursing units, and all other major inventory locations (e.g., operating room, cath lab, and radiology), but only the storeroom and nursing units are maintained routinely. Finally, at Level VI, perpetual inventory is in place and routinely maintained at all inventory locations.

| Stock-Outs: Level VI | *Fewer than 100 stock-outs occur in the hospital annually.* |

Stock-outs—i.e., running out of needed supplies—occur for many reasons. Some, like shortages of manufacturing materials and weather events, are beyond the organization's control, but others are within its control. The goal is to have as few stock-outs as possible. In the CQO framework, performance levels are measured by the number of stock-outs occurring annually. Accordingly, a Level I organization experiences more than 1,000 stock-outs in a year. The number drops to fewer than 800 at Level II, fewer than 600 at Level III, fewer than 400 at Level IV, fewer than 200 at Level V, and fewer than 100 at Level VI.

| Unvalued Inventory: Level VI | *There is no unvalued inventory in any department or location.* |

Unvalued inventory is inventory not captured in the organization's financial records. When this occurs, it distorts the organization's income statement and various key financial indicators such as current assets, working capital, and current ratio.[38] In the CQO framework, Level I organizations have unvalued inventory throughout the organization, but subsequent levels reflect gradually lower levels of unvalued inventory. For example, at Level IV, unvalued inventory is more than 25%, but less than 50% of total stock in any department or location; unvalued inventory is more than 10%, but less than 25% of total stock at Level V. There is no unvalued inventory in any department or location at Level VI.

Purchasing

Purchasing is obviously a core component of CQO given its direct impact on cost. Two purchasing attributes—**electronic data interchange (EDI)** and price/quantity matching—are hallmarks of purchasing/procurement operations in today's environment.

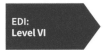

EDI:
Level VI

An EDI system is in place and is used for the purchase of at least 75% of all items, representing at least 85% of all purchase lines and 70% of total spend purchased.

EDI involves "the computer-to-computer exchange of business documents in a standard electronic format between business partners."[39] In healthcare organizations, this means that procurement transactions conducted between the organization and suppliers are computer based, thereby reducing paperwork, eliminating errors associated with paperwork, providing reliable tracking, improving the speed of the ordering process, and, most importantly, transitioning the supply chain from a transactional state to a more strategic model.

There is no EDI system in place in Level I organizations; however, in

---

[38] H. Averkamp, "What Is Inventory Valuation?" AccountingCoach®, accessed August 7, 2014, http://www.accountingcoach.com/blog/what-is-inventory-valuation.

[39] "What is EDI (Electronic Data Interchange)?" EDI Basics, accessed August 6, 2014, http://www.edibasics.com/what-is-edi/.

succeeding levels, the system is used for increasing amounts of purchased items. For example, at Level II, the EDI system is used for most items purchased through the prime distributors (med/surg and lab) only and represents up to 35% of all purchase lines and 10% of total spend purchased. At Level III, an EDI system is used for most items purchased through the prime distributors and up to 25% of all other items while representing up to 45% of all purchase lines and 20% of total spend purchased. At Level IV, the EDI system is used for most or all items purchased through prime distributors (med/surg and lab) and up to 35% of all other items; it represents 55% of all purchase lines and 40% of total spend purchased. At Level V, an EDI system is used for most or all items purchased through prime distributors and up to 50% of all other items; it represents up to 75% of all purchase lines and 50% of total spend purchased. Finally, at Level VI, the EDI system is used for the purchase of at least 75% of all items, representing at least 85% of all purchase lines and 70% of total spend purchased.

Price/Quantity Matching: Level VI

There is electronic three- to five-way price/quantity matching (contract→P.O→receipt→invoice→reimbursement reconciliation) performed on all items, representing up to 85% of all purchase lines and 70% of total spend purchased.

There is no price/quantity matching (manual or electronic) at Level I. At Level II, there is manual three-way price/quantity matching (P.O.→receipt→invoice), but this occurs sporadically (e.g., when there is a payment issue with a supplier). Level III organizations have electronic three-way price/quantity matching, but only for selected vendors or items, capturing only up to 35% of all purchase lines and 10% of total spend. At Level IV, there is electronic three-way price/quantity matching for all vendors or items, representing up to 50% of all purchase lines and 35% of total spend purchased. Four-way price/quantity matching (contract→P.O.→receipt→invoice reconciliation) is characteristic of most Level V organizations, and it represents up to 75% of all purchase lines and 50% of total spend purchased. Finally, Level VI organizations have five-way price matching (contract→P.O.→receipt→invoice→reimbursement reconciliation), which is performed on items equaling up to 85% of all purchase lines and 70% of total spend.

Receiving

The receiving department is the organization's designated location where purchases are initially delivered. This department is typically responsible for order receipt and verification, record keeping, order status tracking, distribution management and/or coordination, and related activities, all of which are important for managing and controlling costs. For receiving, the CQO framework distinguishes between stock and non-stock items, where stock items are patient care supplies, etc., that must be available continuously and are maintained in inventory, while non-stock items are usually one-time or infrequent purchases that don't require storage or regular replenishment.

> **Receiving–Stock Purchases: Level VI**
>
> *All deliveries are received at a loading dock and loaded into the MMIS system via handhelds; there is a regular timetable for sending items to storerooms; most items are received from a coordinated distributor prepackaged for delivery to storeroom inventory locations.*

In a Level I organization, there is no central receiving function for either stock or non-stock purchases. Deliveries of stock items at all subsequent levels are received at the loading dock. They are tracked via a paper process at Level II, entered into the MMIS manually at Level III, and entered into the MMIS via handhelds at Levels IV, V, and VI. Additionally, at Level V, many items are received from the distributor prepackaged for delivery to storeroom inventory locations, but there is no regular timetable for sending items to storerooms. At Level VI, most items are received from the distributor prepackaged for delivery to storeroom inventory locations, and there is a regular timetable for sending items to storerooms.

> **Receiving–Non-Stock Purchases: Level VI**
>
> *There is a centralized process in place for receiving non-stock purchases, which is adhered to by all departments/service lines.*

With respect to **non-stock purchases**, Level II organizations are depicted by a centralized receiving process, but adherence by departments/service lines is sporadic. At subsequent levels, compliance with the centralized receiving process by departments/service lines gradually increases from at least 25% (Level III) to at least 50% (Level IV) to at least 75% (Level V) to all departments/service lines (Level VI).

Reimbursement

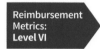

Supply cost and revenue metrics are continuously captured and tracked; information is routinely used to support decision making enterprise-wide.

The ability to link supply costs and reimbursement is a basic cornerstone of the CQO framework. Put simply, organizations must be able to determine their supply costs and how they are reimbursed for their supply purchases.

At Level I, there is little or no information that enables institutions to accurately determine their supply costs and/or their reimbursement for supplies. At the other end of the spectrum (Level VI), supply costs and revenue metrics are continuously captured and tracked, and this information is used routinely to support decision making enterprise-wide. Levels II–V reflect successive degrees of performance in this critical arena. Specifically, supply-related cost and revenue data are used to evaluate against benchmarks for such high-level purposes as total budget and labor costs at Level II; select departments use supply-related cost and revenue data on a regular basis at Level III; high-level supply cost and revenue metrics and basic dashboards have been developed and are available for use at Level IV; and, at Level V, supply cost and revenue metrics are continuously captured and tracked with the information used periodically (but not routinely as in Level VI) to support decision making.

Requisitioning

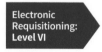

An electronic requisitioning system is used by at least 90% of all departments and service lines and represents at least 75% of all purchase lines and 65% of total spend purchased.

Electronic requisitioning is a must for healthcare organizations in today's world. Automating the requisitioning process offers numerous benefits, including improving accuracy, streamlining the approval process, facilitating order tracking, quantifying demand, eliminating transactional processes, and so forth.

- In Level I organizations, all requisitioning is performed manually.
- Electronic requisitioning is introduced at Level II, where it is used by at least 10% of all departments and service lines and represents 5% of all purchase lines and 5% of total spend purchased.
- At Level III, use of electronic requisitioning encompasses at least 25% of all departments and service lines and represents up to 15% of all purchase lines and 10% of total spend.
- At Level IV, electronic requisitioning is used by at least 50% of all departments and service lines, constituting 35% of all purchase lines and 30% of total spend purchased.
- Level V is characterized by the use of electronic requisitioning by at least 75% of all departments and service lines, reflecting up to 50% of all purchase lines and 40% of total spend purchased.
- Finally, Level VI organizations are those in which electronic requisitioning is used almost universally (defined in the CQO framework as used by at least 90% of all departments and service lines, representing at least 75% of all purchase lines and 65% of total spend purchased).

Advancing from Level I to Level VI in this arena involves first and foremost the purchase and installation of an electronic requisitioning solution. There are many such solutions on the market; some are limited only to the requisitioning process while others embed requisitioning within a broader set of features and functionality (e.g., receiving, EDI, inventory management, etc.) that are constantly evolving and being enhanced. Deployment throughout the organization is the ultimate goal, and achieving it requires significant changes in management efforts; ongoing end-user education and support; supplier linkages and buy-in, where possible; and other such efforts.[40]

---

[40] *Best Practices in e-Procurement: Reducing Costs and Increasing Value Through On-line Buying* (Boston, MA: The Aberdeen Group, December 2005), http://www.purchasing.upenn.edu/news/ag_bpe_0512.pdf.

Value Analysis

Value Analysis is a formal, systematic, evidence-based process for evaluating healthcare products and services for their clinical quality and cost-effectiveness. At its best, this process involves multidisciplinary teams of clinicians and administrators often led by physicians, paying particular attention to physician and clinical preference items. According to the Association of Healthcare Value Analysis Professionals, the average healthcare organization uses between 5,000 and 17,000 products, services, and technologies in any given year.[41] Thus, the goal of value analysis is to ensure that the institution is using products and supplies with demonstrated clinical effectiveness and getting the best possible price for these products and supplies through evaluation, standardization, and other such strategies.

In the CQO framework, value analysis is measured by four attributes: hospital culture; executive oversight; introduction of new clinical and non-clinical products, services, and technology; and continuous intersection of cost, quality, and outcomes.

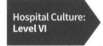
Hospital Culture: Level VI

There is an enterprise-wide CQO culture and focus, with the supply chain owning the intersection of cost, quality, and outcomes.

On the hospital culture front, there are no value analysis initiatives in a Level I organization. At Level II, supply chain, finance, operations, and clinical staff recognize the need for value analysis, but operate independently. At Level III, operations and clinical staff focus primarily on quality and outcomes, while finance and supply chain focus on cost. At Level IV, perspectives begin to merge with operations and clinical staff focusing on quality and outcomes in select clinical areas with some involvement from supply chain staff. Level V organizations are exemplified by an interdisciplinary culture that supports the integration of the supply chain and cost reduction within clinical operations. At Level VI, there is an enterprise-wide CQO

---

[41] "Statement of Purpose," Association of Healthcare Value Analysis Professionals (AHVAP), accessed August 7, 2014, http://www.ahvap.org/?page=Statement_of_Purpose.

culture and focus with supply chain owning the intersection of cost, quality, and outcomes.

Executive Oversight: Level VI

There is a physician-led Value Analysis Steering Committee with participation from all key stakeholders (e.g., finance, supply chain, performance improvement, and clinical).

Executive oversight is essential for an effective value analysis program. In Level I organizations, there is little or no executive oversight of cost reduction or supply chain–related activities. At Level II, there is executive oversight, but it is limited to major initiatives. Supply chain leadership emerges in Level III organizations, whereby products are evaluated for cost and clinical evaluations are included. At Level IV, supply chain leadership, in collaboration with physicians, tackle cost reduction or other supply chain–related initiatives. In Level V organizations, there is a physician-led Value Analysis Steering Committee with rotational physician team members. And, at Level VI, a physician-led Value Analysis Steering Committee is established and involves all key stakeholders (e.g., finance, supply chain, performance improvement, and clinical).

New Products, Services, Technology: Level VI

More than 75% of new products, services, and technology are evaluated by an inter-departmental committee and, if selected, are tested for clinical effectiveness by a technology committee.

New products, services, and technology are adopted by Level I organizations without any formal evaluation process. At Level II, the evaluation of new technology is department specific. The remaining performance levels are characterized by a successive number of products, services, and technology subject to a formal evaluation process by an interdepartmental committee prior to purchase. Thus, fewer than 25% of new products are formally evaluated at Level III, 25%–50% are formally evaluated at Level IV, 50%–75% are evaluated at Level V, and more than 75% are evaluated by a formal value analysis process and the Value Analysis Steering Committee at Level VI.

| Continuous Intersection of Cost, Quality, Outcomes: **Level VI** | ***All initiatives are evidence-, outcome-, quality-, service-, reimbursement-, and cost-based, and are continuously reviewed.*** |

With respect to the intersection of CQO, there are no cost-, quality-, or outcomes-driven initiatives in any department, service line, or enterprise-wide in Level I organizations. In Level II organizations, these initiatives are sporadic. At Level III, there are the beginnings of moderate integration of these initiatives across departments/service lines. At Level IV, there is significant integration between cost-, quality-, and outcome-driven initiatives across departments/service lines. At Level V, there is an enterprise-wide continuous process of establishing cost, quality-, and outcome-driven initiatives. Finally, at Level VI, all initiatives are evidence-, outcomes-, quality-, service-, reimbursement-, and cost-based, and they are continuously reviewed.

Conclusion

The ever-increasing pressure on hospitals and health systems to reduce costs while improving quality and outcomes gave rise to the CQO Movement, which, for the first time, explicitly recognizes the major impact that supply chain operations have on cost, quality, and outcomes, and provides a conceptual framework and systematic approach to supply chain improvement. What is becoming clear, however, is that hospital and health system executives need strategic support from the healthcare supply chain to achieve a larger, related goal: healthcare's Triple Aim. The three dimensions of the Triple Aim are:

- improving the patient experience of care (including quality and satisfaction);
- improving the health of populations; and
- reducing the per capita cost of healthcare.

For hospitals/health systems that embrace the CQO Movement, the supply chain goal is attaining Level VI—within each focus area and overall.

Achieving this goal requires strong leadership by supply chain executives, solid commitment and support from the uppermost levels of management, and the buy-in and participation of clinicians and administrators in every corner of the organization.

The ultimate goal for hospitals and health systems, however, is to use the CQO framework as part of a *continuous improvement process toward the Triple Aim*. The Triple Aim requires ambitious improvement at all levels of a health system, which is why taking a systematic approach to deriving greater value from existing inputs and resources is critical. As no one person or department within a hospital is accountable for all dimensions of the Triple Aim, the facilitator role that supply chain can play while sitting at the intersection of cost, quality, and outcomes becomes essential to addressing these goals.

For most hospitals/health systems, change will be incremental, with improvements building one upon another and coming in successive steps. CQO is a journey, one that will be defined by myriad factors, including organizational complexities, resources, and both known as well as unknown externalities. This book and the accompanying Hospital Supply Chain Performance Self-Assessment are tools to be used to guide that journey and support hospitals and health systems in their efforts to develop and maintain supply chains that perform at top levels.

Appendix A: Methods

The Hospital Supply Chain Performance Self-Assessment™ ("Self-Assessment") was developed to help hospital/health system leaders evaluate the performance of their supply chain operations. For purposes of this Self-Assessment, "supply chain operations" is defined to include twelve "focus areas" and their associated attributes, as follows:

FOCUS AREAS (in alphabetical order)	ATTRIBUTES
Continuous Process Improvement	CPI Process, Procedures, and Technology
Contracting	▸ Centralized, Enterprise-wide Contracting Control and Purchasing ▸ GPO Contracting ▸ Local Contracting
Data Management	▸ Item Master File ▸ Reporting ▸ Charge Capture
Distribution	Distribution Schedule
Education and Training	Supply Chain Education
Internal Controls	Controls
Inventory Management	▸ Perpetual Inventory ▸ PAR Levels ▸ Cycle Counting ▸ Charge to Order System ▸ Unvalued Inventory ▸ Inventory Delivery Systems ▸ Stock-outs ▸ Inventory Turns
Purchasing	▸ EDI ▸ Five-Way Price/Quantity Matching
Receiving	▸ Stock Purchases ▸ Non-stock Purchases
Reimbursement	Metrics
Requisitioning	Electronic Requisitioning
Value Analysis	▸ Hospital Culture ▸ Executive Oversight ▸ Introduction of New Clinical and Non-clinical Products, Services, and Technology ▸ Continuous Intersection of Cost, Quality, and Outcomes

Each attribute was further broken into six specific successive levels of performance ("performance levels"), such that Level I represents the lowest level of performance for the specified attribute and Level VI represents optimal performance for that attribute. Taken together, the focus areas, attributes, and performance levels comprise a proprietary matrix that forms the basis of the Self-Assessment.

Hospital/Health System Unique Identifiers

Each Self-Assessment respondent is assigned a unique identifier ("Self-Assessment Unique ID") consisting of a 12-character code, as follows:

- **SS:** two letters for the state
- **YYY:** three digits for the health system
  (where there is no health system, this field = 000)
- **HHHH:** four digits for the hospital
- **RRR:** three digits for the respondent (by title)

The first three elements of the Self-Assessment Unique ID (*state, health system, hospital*) are captured in a specially designed lookup table, which was derived from a proprietary algorithm developed by the Health Economics, Finance, and Outcomes Research division of the Greater New York Hospital Association (GNYHA). The last element of the Self-Assessment Unique ID (*respondent by title*) reflects more than 100 hospital/health system administrative and clinical titles assigned unique values. While all data will be kept confidential and reported only in the aggregate, this ID system enables Self-Assessment responses from within the same hospital, across hospitals within the same health system, and over different time periods to be linked and analyzed together.

Weighting the Focus Areas

Recognizing that individual focus areas are not likely to have equal impact on cost, quality, and outcomes, relative weights were developed. The weights were derived from an opinion survey conducted in July 2013 of chief operating officers, chief financial officers, and supply chain executives in GNYHA member hospitals.[42] The survey asked respondents to rate on a five-point scale[43] how important each focus area is in affecting hospital costs, quality, and outcomes. The vast majority of respondents ranked each focus area as either "Extremely Important" or "Very Important" (followed by "Important" to a lesser degree). Fewer than 5% of all responses ranked any of the focus areas as "Not Important" or "Somewhat Important." To compute weights in view of this distribution of responses, the "Extremely Important" and "Very Important" responses for each focus area were combined, summed across all focus areas (N = 481), and normalized to equal 100. The value of the combined "Extremely Important/ Very Important" responses for each focus area was then computed in percentage terms, yielding the following weights:

FOCUS AREA	WEIGHT
Continuous Process Improvement	8.9
Contracting	10.2
Data Management	10.4
Distribution	6.0
Education and Training	8.1
Internal Controls	10
Inventory Management	8.5
Purchasing	10.0
Receiving	3.3
Reimbursement	8.9
Requisitioning	5.4
Value Analysis	10.2

Computing Self-Assessment Scores

The Self-Assessment tool generates a raw (unweighted) score for each focus area and an overall weighted composite score. For focus areas with more than one attribute, the average of all attributes is calculated. Individual focus area scores range from 1 to 6 (up to one decimal point). The overall composite score

---

[42] Response rate = 22%.
[43] Not Important, Somewhat Important, Important, Very Important, Extremely Important.

is calculated by multiplying the individual focus area raw score by the weight for that focus area, summing all the weighted focus area scores, and dividing 100 by the sum of the weighted scores. Overall composite scores range from 1 to 6 (up to two decimal points). Multiple responses from the same hospital/ health system are averaged, thereby producing an average score for each focus area and an average overall composite score.

NOTE	No individual respondent results are reported unless only one assessment is completed by a hospital/health system.

The Hospital Supply Chain Performance Self-Assessment™: An Online Tool

The Self-Assessment is an online tool developed in collaboration with IKM, an internationally recognized company specializing in knowledge measurement solutions and services including assessments, certifications, software applications, and consulting services. The Self-Assessment is adapted from IKM's web-based assessment products. IKM provided special programming and support in a number of areas, including customized assessment templates, report design, scoring, automated replies and reminders, and more. IKM also provides secure data hosting services for this project.

Scheduling the Self-Assessment

Self-Assessments are scheduled by the performance improvement team at Nexera. Once scheduled, respondents receive a link to the Self-Assessment and have up to thirty days to complete it. Each time a hospital/health system is interested in repeating the assessment, a new assessment is scheduled so that results can be reported for individual time periods and compared over time. Repeating the assessment at periodic intervals (e.g., every six months or annually) enables a hospital/health system to track changes and obtain feedback about supply chain operations to inform future performance improvement efforts.

To schedule a Self-Assessment for your institution, contact Nexera, Inc., at **nexerainc.com** *or www.nexerainc.com/CQOAssessment.*

Appendix B: Healthcare Terms

ABC Analysis

A classification of items in an inventory according to importance defined in terms of criteria such as sales volume and purchase volume.[1]

Absorption Costing

In cost management, an approach to inventory valuation in which variable costs and a portion of fixed costs are assigned to each unit of production. The fixed costs are usually allocated to units of output on the basis of direct labor hours, machine hours, or material costs. **Synonym: Allocation Costing.**[1]

Accessorial Charges

A carrier's charge for accessorial services such as loading, unloading, pickup, and delivery, or any other charge deemed appropriate.[1]

Accounts Payable (A/P)

The value of goods and services acquired for which payment has not yet been made.[1]

Accounts Receivable (A/R)

The value of goods shipped or services rendered to a customer for whom payment has not been received. Usually includes an allowance for bad debts.[1]

Activity

Work performed by people, equipment, technologies, or facilities. Activities are usually described by the action-verb-adjective-noun grammar convention. Activities may occur in a linked sequence and activity-to-activity assignments may exist. In activity-based cost accounting, a task or activity, performed by or at a resource, required in producing the organization's output of goods and services. A resource may be a person, machine, or facility. Activities are grouped into pools by type of activity and allocated to products. In project management, an element of work on a project. It usually has an anticipated duration, anticipated cost, and expected resource requirements. Sometimes major activity is used for larger bodies of work.[1]

Activity-Based Budgeting (ABB)

An approach to budgeting where a company uses an understanding of its activities and driver relationships to quantitatively estimate workload and resource requirements as part of an ongoing business plan. Budgets show the types, number of, and cost of resources that activities are expected to consume based on forecasted workloads. The budget is part of an organization's activity-based planning process and can be used in evaluating its success in setting and pursuing strategic goals.[1]

Activity-Based Costing (ABC)

A methodology that measures the cost and performance of cost objects, activities, and resources. Cost objects consume activities, and activities consume resources. Resource costs are assigned to activities based on their use of those resources, and activity costs are reassigned to cost objects (outputs) based on the cost objects' proportional use of those activities. Activity-based costing incorporates causal relationships between cost objects and activities and between activities and resources.[1]

Actual Costs

The labor, material, and associated overhead costs charged against a job as it moves through the production process.[1]

Accountable Care Organization (ACO)

An entity, usually comprising hospitals, physicians, and other providers, that takes responsibility for the healthcare needs of a defined population. The providers within the ACO typically continue to bill fee-for-service, but they then share in savings achieved relative to a spending benchmark or an expected spending amount. The Medicare Shared Savings Program established in the

Affordable Care Act allows ACOs to contract with Medicare to share in cost reductions realized by investing in infrastructure and redesigning the care process while meeting quality-of-care performance standards for an assigned population of Medicare beneficiaries. *See Affordable Care Act.*[22]

Acute Care

Healthcare delivered to patients experiencing an illness or health problem of a short-term or episodic nature. This term is used in contrast to the term "continuing care," which is often used to describe nursing homes or home healthcare.[2]

Advance Material Request

Ordering materials before the release of the formal product design. This early release is required because of long lead times.[1]

Adverse Event

In the context of healthcare, an injury or an unfavorable and/or unanticipated outcome experienced by a patient, resulting from a medical intervention. Not all adverse events are medical errors.[2]

Affordable Care Act (ACA)

The comprehensive health reform legislation signed by President Obama in March 2010, designed to extend health insurance coverage to an additional 32 million Americans while reforming the healthcare delivery system to reduce the rate of growth in healthcare costs over time. The ACA creates state health exchanges through which lower-income Americans can purchase qualified health insurance plans with federal subsidies, beginning in 2014, and also expands Medicaid to cover all Americans with income below 133% of the federal poverty level. The ACA mandates that most Americans have health insurance beginning in 2014 or pay a modest penalty, and it imposes penalties on large employers that do not provide health insurance for their employees. Certain insurance company practices, such as denying coverage due to preexisting conditions, are prohibited. The subsidies and Medicaid expansions are financed through Medicare and Medicaid cuts to healthcare providers, as well as tax increases on high-income earners, insurance companies, medical devices, and others. Delivery system and payment reforms include Medicare penalties for hospital readmissions, bundled payment pilot programs, the creation of accountable care organizations, value-based purchasing programs, and others. *See Accountable Care Organizations (ACO).*[2]

Air Cargo
Freight moved by air transportation.[1]

Allocation
A distribution of costs using calculations that may be unrelated to physical observations or direct or repeatable cause-and-effect relationships. Because of the arbitrary nature of allocations, costs based on cost causal assignment are viewed as more relevant for management decision-making. Allocation of available inventory to customer and production orders.[1]

Ambulatory Payment Classification (APC)
Medicare's payment classification system to reimburse hospitals for outpatient services under the outpatient prospective payment system. Each APC comprises services that are comparable both clinically and with respect to resource utilization.[2]

American National Standards Institute (ANSI)
A nonprofit organization chartered to develop, maintain, and promulgate voluntary US national standards in a number of areas, especially with regard to setting EDI standards. ANSI is the US representative to the International Standards Organization (ISO).[1]

American Society for Quality (ASQ)
Founded in 1946, a not-for-profit educational organization consisting of 144,000 members who are interested in quality improvement.[1]

Anti-Kickback Law

A 1972 federal law stating that anyone who knowingly and willfully receives or pays anything of value to influence the referral of federal healthcare program business, including Medicare and Medicaid, can be held accountable for a felony. Violations of the law are punishable by up to five years in prison, criminal fines up to $25,000, administrative civil money penalties up to $50,000, and exclusion from participation in federal healthcare programs. The Affordable Care Act amended aspects of the Anti-Kickback Law, most notably establishing that a violation of the Anti-Kickback Law constitutes a false claim for purposes of the Federal False Claims Act. Because concerns arose among healthcare providers that the law's broad scope might prohibit some relatively innocuous—and in some cases even beneficial—arrangements, Congress in 1987 authorized the US Department of Health and Human Services to issue regulations designating specific "safe harbors" for various payment and business practices that, while potentially prohibited by the Anti-Kickback Law, would not be prosecuted.[2]

Available to Promise (ATP)

The uncommitted portion of a company's inventory and planned production maintained in the master schedule to support customer-order promising. The ATP quantity is the uncommitted inventory balance in the first period and is normally calculated for each period in which a master production scheduling receipt is scheduled. In the first period, ATP includes on-hand inventory less customer orders that are due and overdue. Three methods of calculation are used: discrete ATP, cumulative ATP with look-ahead, and cumulative ATP without look-ahead.[1]

Average Cost

Total cost, fixed plus variable, divided by total output.[1]

Back Order

Product ordered but out of stock and promised to ship when the product becomes available.[1]

Balanced Scorecard

A structured measurement system based on a mix of financial and nonfinancial measures of business performance. A list of financial and operational measurements used to evaluate organizational or supply chain performance. The dimensions of the balanced scorecard may include customer perspective, business process perspective, financial perspective, and innovation and learning perspectives. It formally connects overall objectives, strategies, and measurements. Each dimension has goals and measurements. *See Scorecard.*[1]

Bar Code

A symbol consisting of a series of printed bars representing values. A system of optical characters for scanning and tracking units by reading a series of printed bars for translation into a numeric or alphanumeric identification code. A popular example is the UPC code used on retail packaging.[1]

Basing-Point Pricing

A pricing system in which the buyer pays a base price plus a set shipping price depending on the distance from a specific location. The basing point pricing system sets a predetermined location, known as the basing point, then adds a transportation charge depending on how far away the buyer is from that location. Typically, the basing point is the same location as the manufacturing point, and the shipping charge is determined despite the actual location of the buyer or seller.[3]

Benchmarking

The process of comparing performance against the practices of other leading companies for the purpose of improving performance. Companies also benchmark internally by tracking and comparing current performance with past performance.[1]

Benefit-Cost Ratio

An analytical tool used in public planning; a ratio of total measurable benefits divided by the initial capital cost.[1]

Best Practice

A specific process or group of processes that have been recognized as the best method for conducting an action. Best practices may vary by industry or geography depending on the environment being used. Best-practices methodology may be applied with respect to resources, activities, cost object, or processes.[1]

Best-Unit-of-Measure (BUM) Distribution

See Low-Unit-of-Measure (LUM) Distribution.

Billing

A carrier terminal activity that determines the proper rate and total charges for a shipment and issues a freight bill.[1]

Bill of Lading (BOL)

A transportation document that is the contract of carriage, containing the terms and conditions between the shipper and carrier.[1]

Bill of Material (BOM)

A structured list of all the materials or parts and quantities needed to produce a particular finished product, assembly, subassembly, or manufactured part, whether purchased or not.[1]

Blanket Purchase Order

A long-term commitment to a supplier for material against which short-term releases will be generated to satisfy requirements. Oftentimes, blanket orders cover only one item with predetermined delivery dates.[1]

Break-Even Point

The level of production or the volume of sales at which operations are neither profitable nor unprofitable. The break-even point is the intersection of the total revenue and total cost curves.[1]

Bundle (Quality Improvement)

A group of evidence-based interventions related to a disease or care process that, when executed together, result in better outcomes than when implemented individually.[2]

Bundled Payments (Finance)

In the context of healthcare financing, 1) a form of payment in which a single payment covers a full episode of care across multiple providers, and 2) the practice of grouping a number of services together and paying a single fee for the group instead of a fee for each service such as a diagnosis-related payment. The Affordable Care Act authorizes Medicare and Medicaid to pilot bundling approaches as a way to improve efficiency. These pilots will explore bundling hospital and physician payments in an acute stay; all acute and post-acute services; and all post-acute services, among other models. *See Affordable Care Act (ACA); Diagnosis-Related Group (DRG).*[2]

Burn Rate

The rate of consumption of cash in a business. Used to determine cash requirements on an ongoing basis. A burn rate of $50,000 would mean the company spends $50,000 a month above any incoming cash flow to sustain its business. Entrepreneurial companies will calculate their burn rate to understand how much time they have before they need to raise more money or show a positive cash flow.[1]

Business Logistics

The process of planning, implementing, and controlling the efficient, effective flow and storage of goods, services, and related information from the point of origin to the point of consumption for the purpose of conforming to customer requirements.[1]

Business Plan

A statement of long-range strategy and revenue, cost, and profit objectives usually accompanied by budgets, a projected balance sheet, and a cash flow (source and application of funds) statement. A business plan is usually stated in terms of dollars and grouped by product family. The business plan is then translated into synchronized tactical functional plans through the production-planning process (or the sales and operations-planning process). Although frequently stated in different terms (dollars versus units), these tactical plans should agree with one another and with the business plan. A document consisting of the business details (organization, strategy, and financing tactics) prepared by an entrepreneur to plan for a new business.[1]

Buyer

An enterprise that arranges for the acquisition of goods or services and agrees to payment terms for such goods or services.[1]

Carve-Out

In the context of healthcare, 1) an arrangement in which a health benefit is provided, managed, and/or paid separately from other benefits, the most prominent examples being mental health, dental, pharmacy, laboratory, and radiology services, and 2) the removal of a portion of the premium that would normally be paid to a health maintenance organization (HMO), and payment of the funds to the entity incurring the cost that the carved-out funds were intended to cover.[2]

Case-Mix Adjustment

Healthcare facilities often seek to evaluate their performance on particular outcomes by comparing their own outcomes with those of one or more facilities. Unadjusted outcomes are generally considered noncomparable because facilities treat patients with different risk factors. To render outcomes more comparable, they can be case-mix adjusted by dividing the outcomes of two or more facilities by their respective case-mix indices (CMI). The CMIs are computed using Medicare, all-payer, or all-patient refined diagnosis-related groups. *See Case-Mix Index (CMI); Diagnosis-Related Group (DRG).*[2]

Case-Mix Index (CMI)

A measure of the severity or resource intensity of the cases in a healthcare facility. A facility's CMI, along with the total number of discharges for a given period and the facility's base rate of payment, can be used to develop a reasonable estimate of anticipated revenue for a given period. The CMI is also used as a planning tool for estimating resources needed to provide care.[2]

Case Rate

A single fee paid for all services associated with a particular illness or "episode" of care. One common episode for which a global fee is paid is obstetrics, where the fee covers prenatal visits, the delivery, and a certain number of postnatal visits. *See Bundled Payments.*[2]

Centers for Medicare & Medicaid Services (CMS)

Federal agency within the Department of Health and Human Services (HHS) responsible for the Medicare and Medicaid programs.[2]

Center for Medicare & Medicaid Innovation (CMMI)

An agency within the Centers for Medicare & Medicaid Services created by the Affordable Care Act to test innovative Medicare and Medicaid payment models. CMMI was granted broad authority to waive sections of law to test different approaches to service delivery and was also given the authority to expeditiously expand successful demonstration projects and pilots nationwide. *See Affordable Care Act (ACA).*[2]

Certified Supplier

A status awarded to a supplier who consistently meets predetermined quality, cost, delivery, financial, and count objectives. Incoming inspection may not be required.[1]

Change Management

The business process that coordinates and monitors all changes to the business processes and applications operated by the business as well as to their internal equipment, resources, operating systems, and procedures. The change management discipline is carried out in a way that minimizes the risk of problems that will affect the operating environment and service delivery to the users.[1]

Charge Description Master (CDM) or Chargemaster

The CDM is a master price list of supplies, devices, medications, services, procedures, and other items for which a distinct charge to the patient exists. It is a financial management form that contains information about the organization's charges for the healthcare services it provides to patients. The CDM collects information on all the goods and services the organization provides to its patients.[4]

Clinical Preference Item (CPI)

Any patient care item or medical device for which a physician, nurse, or other clinician could reasonably be expected to express a product preference compared with similar product(s) available from alternative supplier(s); in contrast with a *commodity* item, where similar products are more likely to be viewed by the physician, nurse, or other clinician as functional equivalents of one another. *See Physician Preference Item (PPI).*[2]

Commodity Procurement Strategy

The purchasing plan for a family of items. This would include the plan to manage the supplier base and solve problems.[1]

Community Benefit

Hospitals' tax-exempt status is generally assessed under the Internal Revenue Service's (IRS) "community benefit" standard. This standard, established by the IRS in a 1969 Revenue Ruling, is a facts and circumstances test that examines whether the hospital takes certain steps to benefit the community, including whether it has an emergency room open to all regardless of ability to pay and whether it admits patients regardless of payer (i.e., does not discriminate against Medicare and Medicaid patients). Congress and others have scrutinized the community benefit standard over the past decade, but it remains intact. It was augmented to some extent by the Affordable Care Act, which requires hospitals to take steps—maintaining written financial assistance and emergency medical policies, conducting community health needs assessments, curtailing certain billing and collection practices, and limiting charges—to remain tax-exempt. In addition, "community benefit" is often used to denote a planned, managed, organized, and measured approach to a healthcare organization's effort in meeting identified community health needs. This interpretation was adopted in principle by the IRS for hospital reporting on the revised IRS Form 990, Schedule H. "Community benefit" implies collaboration with the community to benefit residents—particularly the poor, certain minorities, and other underserved groups—by improving health status and quality of life. Not-for-profit hospitals had to start identifying and quantifying community benefit in tax year 2009 for returns filed in 2010 using the IRS Form 990, Schedule H.[2]

Company Culture
A system of values, beliefs, and behaviors inherent in a company. To optimize business performance, top management must define and create the necessary culture.[1]

Consignment
A shipment handled by a common carrier. The process of a supplier placing goods at a customer location without receiving payment until after the goods are used or sold. *See Consignment Inventory.*[1]

Consignment Inventory
Goods or products that are paid for when they are sold by the reseller, not at the time they are shipped to the reseller. Goods or products that are owned by the vendor until they are sold to the consumer.[1]

Consumer Price Index (CPI)
A year-to-year variable used to reflect inflationary changes in the general economy.

Contingency Planning

Preparing to deal with calamities (e.g., floods) and noncalamitous situations (e.g., strikes) before they occur.[1]

Continuous Process Improvement (CPI)

See Continuous Quality Improvement (CQI).

Continuous Quality Improvement (CQI)

A continuous process that employs rapid cycles of improvement. The Donabedian model provides three dimensions for the quality of care: 1) the structure, which represents the attributes of settings where care is delivered; 2) the process, or whether or not good medical practices are followed; and 3) the outcome, which is the impact of the care on health status.[4]

Contract

An agreement between two or more competent persons or companies to perform or not to perform specific acts or services or to deliver merchandise. A contract may be oral or written. A purchase order, when accepted by a supplier, becomes a contract. Acceptance may be in writing or by performance unless the purchase order requires acceptance in writing.[1]

Cost and Freight (C&F)

The seller quotes a price that includes the cost of transportation to a specific point. The buyer assumes responsibility for loss and damage and pays for the insurance of the shipment.[1]

Cost Management

The management and control of activities and drivers to calculate accurate product and service costs, improve business processes, eliminate waste, influence cost drivers, and plan operations. The resulting information can be useful in setting and evaluating an organization's strategies.[1]

Cost of Capital

The cost to borrow or invest capital.[1]

Cost, Quality, and Outcomes (CQO)

Cost, Quality, and Outcomes (CQO) Movement refers to the intersection of cost, quality, and outcomes, and a more holistic view of the correlation between cost (expenditures as they relate to supplies, services, and other areas in supply chain control [total cost of ownership—TCO] as well as the total cost of care), quality (patient-centered care aimed at achieving the best possible clinical outcomes), and outcomes (financial reimbursement driven by outstanding clinical care at the appropriate costs) as opposed to viewing each independently.[5]

Cost Shifting

Passing the cost of one group on to another group. For example, when the reimbursement rate received by a provider from a payer does not cover the cost of delivering the service, the provider may try to make up the underpayment by charging more, or shifting costs, to other payers.[2]

Council of Supply Chain Management Professionals (CSCMP)

The CSCMP is a not-for-profit professional business organization consisting of individuals throughout the world who have interests and/or responsibilities in logistics and supply chain management, and the related functions that make up these professions. Its purpose is to enhance the development of the logistics and supply chain management professions by providing these individuals with educational opportunities and relevant information through a variety of programs, services, and activities.[1]

Critical Value Analysis

A modified ABC analysis in which a company assigns a subjective critical value to each item in an inventory.[1]

Current Procedural Terminology (CPT)

A classification system developed by the American Medical Association in which unique codes are assigned to procedures and services (but not diagnoses) performed by providers.[2]

Customer/Order Fulfillment Process

A series of customers' interactions with an organization through the order-filling process, including product/service design, production and delivery, and order stats reporting.[1]

Customer-Supplier Partnership

A long-term relationship between a buyer and a supplier characterized by teamwork and mutual confidence. The supplier is considered an extension of the buyer's organization. The partnership is based on several commitments. The buyer provides long-term contracts and uses fewer suppliers. The supplier implements quality assurance processes so incoming inspections can be minimized. The supplier also helps the buyer reduce costs and improve product and process designs.[1]

Cycle Counting/Inventory

An inventory system where counts are performed continuously, often eliminating the need for an annual overall inventory. It is usually set up so that A items are counted regularly (i.e., every month), B items are counted semiregularly (every quarter or six months), and C items are counted perhaps only once a year.[1]

Cycle Time

The amount of time it takes to complete a business process.[1]

Cycle Time to Process Obsolete and End-of-Life Product Returns for Disposal

The total time to process goods returned as obsolete and end of life to actual disposal. This cycle time includes the time a return product authorization (RPA) is created to the time the RPA is approved, from "product available for pickup" to "product received" and from "product receipt" to "product disposal/recycle."[1]

Dashboard

A performance measurement tool used to capture a summary of the key performance indicators/metrics of a company. Metrics dashboards/scorecards should be easy to read and usually have red, yellow, green indicators to flag when the company is not meeting its metrics targets. Ideally, a dashboard/scoreboard should be cross-functional in nature and include both financial and nonfinancial measures. In addition, scorecards should be reviewed regularly—at least on a monthly basis, and weekly in key functions such as manufacturing and distribution where activities are critical to the success of a company. The dashboards/scorecards philosophy can also be applied to external supply chain partners, such as suppliers, to ensure that their objectives and practices align. **Synonym: Scorecard.**[1]

Delivery Instructions

A document issued to a carrier to pick up goods at a location and deliver them to another location.[1]

Delivery Order

A document issued by the customs broker to the ocean carrier as authority to release the cargo to the appropriate party.[1]

Demand Planning Systems

Systems that assist in the process of identifying, aggregating, and prioritizing all sources of demand for the integrated supply chain of a product of service at the appropriate level, horizon, and interval.[1]

Diagnosis-Related Group (DRG)

A diagnosis-based classification system Medicare and Medicaid use to reimburse hospitals for inpatient costs on a per-discharge basis, regardless of length of stay or actual cost. Three DRG classification systems are currently in use, all of which start with basic DRGs—350 case groupings based solely on principal diagnosis—and then are subdivided to a greater or lesser extent. Medicare DRGs split the basic DRGs into about 460 groupings by subdividing some DRGs based on the presence or absence of comorbidities and complications (CCs); these are used for Medicare reimbursement. All-payer refined DRGs (APR-DRGs) split the basic DRGs into about 1,200 groupings by subdividing DRGs based on four severity-of-illness levels.

Direct Cost

A cost that can be directly traced to a cost object since a direct or repeatable cause-and-effect relationship exists. A direct cost uses a direct assignment or cost causal relationship to transfer costs. *See Indirect Cost.*[1]

Disaster Recovery Planning

Contingency planning specifically related to recovering hardware and software (e.g., data centers, application software, operations, personnel, telecommunications) in information system outages.[1]

Disproportionate Share Hospital (DSH)

A hospital that provides a large amount (or disproportionate share) of uncompensated care and/or care to Medicaid and low-income Medicare beneficiaries. These hospitals receive special payments in recognition of the extra costs incurred in caring for these populations. Medicare DSH (pronounced "dish") payments are made to hospitals in which the Medicaid and low-income Medicare share of patient days is at least 15%.[2]

Distributed Inventory

Inventory that is geographically dispersed. For example, where a company maintains inventory in multiple distribution centers to provide a higher level of customer service.[1]

Distribution

Outbound logistics, from the end of the production line to the end user. The activities associated with the movement of material, usually finished goods or service parts, from the manufacturer to the customer. These activities encompass the functions of transportation, warehousing, inventory control, material handling, order administration, site and location analysis, industrial packaging, data processing, and the communications network necessary for effective management. It includes all activities related to physical distribution, as well as the return of goods to the manufacturer. In many cases, this movement is made through one or more levels of field warehouses. The systematic division of a whole into discrete parts having distinctive characteristics. **Synonym: Physical Distribution.**[1]

Distributor

A business that does not manufacture its own products but purchases and resells these products. Such a business usually maintains a finished goods inventory. **Synonym: Wholesaler.**[1]

Distribution Warehouse

A finished goods warehouse from which a company assembles customer orders.[1]

Drop Ship

To take the title of products but not actually handle, stock, or deliver them (e.g., to have one supplier ship directly to another or to have a supplier ship directly to the buyer's customer).[1]

Durable Medical Equipment (DME)

Equipment that is medically necessary. Appropriate medical care ordered by a physician for an individual's specific use, can withstand repeated use, is primarily and customarily to serve a medical purpose, and generally is not useful to an individual in the absence of an illness or injury. Examples of durable medical equipment are wheelchairs, walkers, and home oxygen equipment.[2]

Early Supplier Involvement (ESI)

The process of involving suppliers early in the product design activity and drawing on their expertise, insights, and knowledge to generate better designs in less time and ones that are easier to manufacture with high quality.[1]

Earnings Before Interest and Taxes (EBIT)

A measure of a company's earning power from ongoing operations, equal to earnings (revenues minus cost of sales, operating expenses, and taxes) before deduction of interest payments and income taxes. Also called operating profit.[1]

Economic Order Quantity (EOQ)

An inventory model that determines how much to order by determining the amount that will meet customer service levels while minimizing total ordering and holding costs.[1]

Economic Value Added (EVA)

A measurement of shareholder value as a company's operating profits after tax, less an appropriate charge for the capital used in creating the profits.[1]

Economy of Scale

A phenomenon whereby larger volumes of production reduce unit cost by distributing fixed costs over a larger quantity.[1]

EDI Interchange

Communication between partners in the form of a structured set of messages and service segments starting with an interchange control header and ending with an interchange control trailer. In the context of X.400 EDI messaging, the contents of the primary body of an EDI message.[1]

EDI Standards

Criteria that define the data content and format requirements for specific business transactions (e.g., purchase orders). Using standard formats allows companies to exchange transactions with multiple trading partners more easily. *See American National Standards Institute.*[1]

EDI Transmission

A functional group of one or more EDI transactions sent to the same location in the same transmission and identified by a functional group header and trailer.[1]

Electronic Data Interchange (EDI)

Intercompany, computer-to-computer transmission of business information in a standard format. For EDI purists, "computer-to-computer" means direct transmission from the originating application program to the receiving or processing application program. An EDI transmission consists only of business data, not any accompanying verbiage or free-form messages. Purists might also contend that a standard format is one approved by a national or international standards organization as opposed to formats developed by industry groups or companies.[1]

Electronic Data Interchange Association (EDIA)

A national body that propagates and controls the use of EDI in a given country. All EDIAs are nonprofit organizations dedicated to encouraging EDI growth.[1]

Electronic Health Record (EHR)

A computer-accessible, interoperable resource of clinical and administrative information pertinent to an individual's health. Information drawn from multiple clinical and administrative sources is used primarily by a broad spectrum of clinical personnel involved in the individual's care, enabling them to deliver and coordinate care and promote wellness.[6]

Electronic Medical Record (EMR)

A computer-accessible resource of medical and administrative information available on an individual, collected from and accessible to providers involved in the individual's care within a single care setting.[6]

Emergency Operations Center (EOC)

A facility or location, also known as a command center, from which the response to a disaster is coordinated. Many healthcare facilities establish their own EOCs staffed with individuals in charge of responding to the disaster. Government entities also create EOCs.[2]

End-of-Life Inventory

Inventory on hand that will satisfy future demand for products no longer in production at a company.[1]

Enterprise Resource Planning (ERP) System

A class of software for planning and managing enterprise-wide the resources needed to take customer orders, ship them, account for them, and replenish all needed goods according to customer orders and forecasts. Often includes electronic commerce with suppliers. Examples of ERP systems are the application suites from SAP, Oracle, PeopleSoft, and others.[1]

ePrescribing

The transmission of prescription or prescription-related information using electronic media and information technology standards among a prescriber, dispenser, pharmacy benefit manager, or health plan to reduce prescription errors and expedite timely fulfillment of prescriptions.[2]

Expediting

Moving shipments through regular channels at an accelerated rate. To take extraordinary action because of an increase in relative priority.[1]

Failure Mode and Effect Analysis (FMEA)

The systematic approach of prospectively examining the design of a process or system for possible ways in which process or system failure can occur. FMEA is a proactive type of analysis used in the engineering industry to design safe systems. Using FMEA, potential failures or problems are anticipated and removed or designed out of the system or process under review. Healthcare providers use this analysis to design safer care processes and systems to minimize ways in which medical errors might occur and to mitigate the effects of system/process failures when they do occur.[2]

Fair Value

The value of the carrier's property; the calculation basis has included original cost minus depreciation, replacement cost, and market value.[1]

False Claims Act, Federal

The federal law that prohibits a person or entity from knowingly presenting, or causing to be presented, a false or fraudulent claim for payment to the federal government. A violation of the False Claims Act results in a mandatory civil penalty of $5,500–$11,000 per claim for all claims made after September 29, 1999, plus "treble damages" or three times the amount of damages suffered by the government. The False Claims Act allows an individual, often referred to as a "whistleblower" or "relator" who knows about a person or entity, who is submitting false claims to bring a *qui tam* lawsuit on behalf of the government, and to share in the damages recovered as a result of the suit. The False Claims Act was enacted during the Civil War, subsequently strengthened in 1986, expanded in 2009, and again in the Affordable Care Act of 2010. It has been used consistently against healthcare providers with respect to claims submitted for Medicare or Medicaid payments.[2]

Federal Emergency Management Agency (FEMA)

The US Department of Homeland Security agency that coordinates emergency responses on behalf of the federal government when a state of emergency is declared. FEMA also reimburses local and state government agencies and certain not-for-profits providing government-like services for eligible, disaster-related losses and costs. Costs eligible for reimbursement include removing debris, emergency response measures and repair, and replacing or restoring disaster-damaged public facilities.[2]

Federally Qualified Health Center (FQHC)

A designation assigned to community-based organizations that provide comprehensive primary care and preventive care in underserved urban and rural communities. Such organizations must also comply with regulations specified under Section 330 of the US Public Health Service Act. The regulations include having a board with a majority of members that are consumers. FQHCs may include community health centers, public housing centers, outpatient health programs funded by the Indian Health Service, and programs serving migrants and the homeless. FQHCs qualify for a cash grant, cost-based reimbursement for their Medicaid patients, and free malpractice coverage under the Federal Tort Claims Act (FTCA). The government also designates a category of health centers as "FQHC Look-Alikes." These health centers receive cost-based reimbursement for their Medicaid services but do not receive malpractice coverage under FTCA or a cash grant.[2]

Fee-for-Service

A method of payment that gives reimbursement, usually in predetermined amounts, when a specific service is provided. Fee-for-service payments occur each time a service is rendered as opposed to capitated payments, which are paid on a regular schedule regardless of whether services were rendered.[2]

Field Finished Goods

Inventory kept at locations outside the four walls of the manufacturing plant (i.e., distribution center or warehouse).[1]

Field Warehouse

A warehouse that stores goods on the goods' owner's property while the goods are under a bona fide public warehouse manager's custody. The owner uses the public warehouse receipts as collateral for a loan.[1]

Fill Rate

The percentage of order items that the picking operation actually found.[1]

Fill Rates by Order

Whether orders are received and released consistently or released from a blanket purchase order, this metric measures the percentage of ship-from-stock orders shipped within 24 hours of order "release." Make-to-stock schedules attempt to time the availability of finished goods to match forecasted customer orders or releases. Orders not shipped within 24 hours due to consolidation but available for shipment within 24 hours are reported separately. In calculating elapsed time for order fill rates, the interval begins at ship release and ends when material is consigned for shipment. **Calculation:** [Number of orders filled from stock shipped within 24 hours or order release]/[Total number of stock orders]. The same concept of fill rates can be applied to order lines and individual products to provide statistics on percentage of lines shipped completely and percentage of products shipped completely.[1]

Final Destination

The last stopping point for a shipment.[1]

Finished Goods Inventory (FG or FGI)

Products completely manufactured, packaged, stored, and ready for distribution.[1]

Four-Wall Inventory

The stock contained within a single facility or building.[1]

Freight

Goods being transported from one place to another.[1]

Fully Allocated Cost

The variable cost associated with a particular output unit, plus a common cost allocation.[1]

Gainsharing

Hospital-physician arrangement in which a hospital gives physicians a percentage share of any reduction in the hospital's costs for patient care attributable in part to the physicians' efforts to improve overall efficiency and quality of care. The Federal Deficit Reduction Act of 2005 required the secretary of the US Department of Health and Human Services to establish a gainsharing demonstration program for up to six projects to test and evaluate methodologies and arrangements between hospitals and physicians to improve the quality and efficiency of care provided to Medicare beneficiaries, and to develop improved operational and financial hospital performance with sharing of gains as specified in the project. Each project had to develop measures to monitor quality and efficiency. The project was authorized for January 1, 2007, through December 31, 2009. The Affordable Care Act extended the project through September 30, 2011. In August 2011, the Center for Medicare and Medicaid Innovation announced a number of bundled payment and shared savings initiatives that would allow many more hospitals to participate in gainsharing programs. *See Bundled Payments.*[2]

Global Location Number (GLN)

The GS1 Identification Key used for any location (physical, operational, or legal) that needs to be identified for use in the supply chain. The GLN is a globally unique number that can be used to access master data about a location.[7]

Goods

A term associated with more than one definition: 1) common term indicating movable property, merchandise, or wares, 2) all materials used to satisfy demands, and 3) all or part of the cargo received from the shipper, including any equipment supplied by the shipper.[1]

Group Purchasing Organization (GPO)

An organization that negotiates volume discount contracts with suppliers on behalf of its member facilities, providing them with favorable pricing, terms and conditions, and other benefits. GPO participants can include hospitals, medical group practices, nursing homes, and other long-term care facilities, surgery centers, managed care organizations, home infusion providers, provider pharmacies, clinics, and integrated delivery networks.[2]

GS1

GS1 is an international not-for-profit association with members in more than one hundred countries. GS1 is dedicated to the design and implementation of global standards and solutions to improve the efficiency and visibility of supply and demand chains globally and across sectors. The GS1 system of standards is the most widely used supply chain standards system in the world.[8]

GS1 Healthcare US

The national healthcare industry user group that supports the adoption and implementation of the GS1 global standards. Its mission is to proactively work with US healthcare providers, manufacturers, distributors, group purchasing organizations, industry associations, pharmacies, and healthcare professionals to implement and effectively use GS1 standards, best practices, and standards-based solutions to improve patient safety and supply chain security and efficiency and to promote accurate cross-referencing of like products.[8]

GTIN

Global Tracking Identification Number or Global Trade Item Number. GTIN is the globally unique EAN.UCC System identification number or key used for trade items (products and services). It is used for uniquely identifying trade items (products and services) sold, delivered, warehoused, and billed throughout the retail and commercial distribution channels. Unlike a UPC number, which only provides information specific to a group of products, the GTIN gives each product its own specific identifying number, giving greater accuracy in tracking.[9]

Handling Costs

Costs involved in moving, transferring, preparing, and otherwise handling inventory.[1]

Healthcare Common Procedural Coding System (HCPCS)

The coding system used by the Medicare program. HCPCS includes Current Procedural Terminology codes and additional codes used mainly by Medicare. *See Current Procedural Terminology (CPT).*[2]

Healthcare Supply Chain Association (HSCA)

Formerly known as the Health Industry Group Purchasing Association (HIGPA), HSCA is a broad-based trade association representing 16 group purchasing organizations, including for-profit and not-for-profit corporations, purchasing groups, associations, multihospital systems, and healthcare provider alliances. HSCA's mission is to advocate on behalf of healthcare group purchasing associations, provide educational opportunities designed to improve efficiencies in the purchase, sale, and use of all goods and services within the health industry, and promote meaningful dialogue among GPOs.[2]

Hospital Incident Command System (HICS)

A form of the incident command system (ICS) healthcare facilities use. A comprehensive management system intended for use in both emergent and nonemergent situations, HICS includes an organizational chart that indicates positions of responsibility, including incident commander and section chiefs (operations, planning, logistics, and financial/administration). The HICS organizational structure outlines roles for various individuals during an emergency and serves as an "all-hazards" approach to management.[2]

Inbound Logistics

The management of materials from suppliers and vendors into production processes or storage facilities.[1]

Indirect Cost

A resource or activity cost that cannot be directly traced to a final cost object since no direct or repeatable cause-and-effect relationship exists. An indirect cost uses an assignment or allocation to transfer cost.[1]

Information System (I/S)

Managing the flow of data in an organization in a systematic, structured way to assist in planning, implementing, and controlling.[1]

Institute for Healthcare Improvement (IHI)

A not-for-profit organization whose goal is to drive health improvement by advancing the quality and value of healthcare. IHI serves as a source of knowledge and best practices to improve healthcare processes and outcomes. Two major IHI campaigns that spurred national quality improvement initiatives were the 100,000 Lives Campaign and the Five Million Lives Campaign, which challenged hospitals to commit to implementing changes in care that have been demonstrated to improve patient outcomes and prevent avoidable deaths.[2]

Integrated Delivery System (IDS)

In the context of healthcare, a group of organizations that collectively provide a full range of health-related services in a coordinated fashion to those who use the system. Some researchers believe an IDS must be fiscally accountable (that is, must share the risk in some way to help control costs).[2]

Inventory

Raw materials, works in process, finished goods, and supplies required for creation of a company's goods and services. The number of units and/or value of the stock of goods held by a company.[1]

Inventory Carrying Cost

One of the elements comprising a company's total supply chain management costs. These costs consist of the following:

Opportunity Cost: The opportunity cost of holding inventory. This should be based on your company's own cost of capital standards using the following formula: **Calculation:** [Cost of Capital]x[Average Net Value of Inventory].

Shrinkage: Costs associated with breakage, pilferage, and deterioration of inventories. Usually pertains to the loss of material through handling damage, theft, or neglect.

Insurance and Taxes: The cost of insuring inventories and taxes associated with the holding of inventory.

Total Obsolescence for Raw Material, WIP, and Finished Goods Inventory: Inventory reserves taken due to obsolescence and scrap, including products exceeding the shelf life (i.e., spoils and is no good for use in its original purpose). Does not include reserves taken for field service parts.

Channel Obsolescence: Aging allowances paid to channel partners, provisions for buy-back agreements, etc. Includes all material that becomes obsolete while in a distribution channel. Usually a distributor will demand a refund on material that goes bad (shelf life) or is no longer needed because of changing needs.

Field Service Parts Obsolescence: Reserves taken due to obsolescence and scrap. Field service parts are inventories kept at locations outside the four walls of the manufacturing plant (i.e., distribution center or warehouse).[1]

Inventory Cost
The cost of holding goods, usually expressed as a percentage of the inventory value; includes the cost of capital, warehousing, taxes, insurance, depreciation, and obsolescence.[1]

Inventory, Days of
The number of days of inventory on hand at any given time.[1]

Inventory In Transit
Inventory in a carrier's possession being transported to the buyer.[1]

Inventory Management

The process of ensuring the availability of products through inventory administration.[1]

Inventory Planning Systems

The systems that help strategically balance inventory policy and customer service levels throughout the supply chain. These systems usually calculate time-phased order quantities and safety stock using selected inventory strategies. Some inventory planning systems conduct what-if analyses and compare the current inventory policy with simulated inventory scenarios to improve the inventory ROI.[1]

Inventory Turns

The cost of goods sold divided by the average level of inventory on hand. This ratio measures how many times a company's inventory has been sold during a period of time. Operationally, inventory turns are measured as total throughput divided by average level of inventory for a given period. How many times a year the average inventory for a firm changes over or is sold.[1]

Item Master File (IMF)

The electronic file that incorporates all items a facility purchases with the item name, item numbers, order quantity, and price. Essential to the purchasing and inventory function, however, it is often left to accounting to manage.[1]

Joint Commission, The (TJC)

A national accrediting and standards-setting body that evaluates and accredits healthcare facilities and programs on a voluntary basis (formerly the Joint Commission on Accreditation of Organizations, or JCAHO). The Joint Commission is an independent not-for-profit organization governed by a board that includes physicians, nurses, and consumers as well as representatives of organizations such as the American Hospital Association. TJC grants accreditation by surveying and evaluating a healthcare organization's performance against a set of standards in areas affecting patient health and safety. Accreditation is often required for affiliation agreements with other healthcare organizations and other contractual or financial arrangements. Under federal law, hospitals accredited by TJC are considered or "deemed" to be in compliance with the Medicare Conditions of Participation, a necessary eligibility requirement to participate in Medicare and Medicaid reimbursement programs. TJC currently provides accreditation for a variety of organizations: ambulatory healthcare, behavioral healthcare, critical access hospitals, home care, hospitals, laboratory services, long-term care, and office-based surgery.[2]

Just-in-Time (JIT)

An inventory control system that controls material flow into assembly and manufacturing plants by coordinating demand and supply to the point where desired materials arrive just in time for use. An inventory reduction strategy, it feeds production lines with products delivered just in time. Developed by the auto industry, it refers to shipping goods in smaller, more frequent lots.[1]

Just-in-Time II (JIT II)

Vendor-managed operations taking place within a customer's facility. JIT II was popularized by the Bose Corporation. The supplier reps, called "inplants," place orders to their own companies, relieving the customer's buyers from this task. Many also become involved at deeper levels, such as participating in new product-development projects and manufacturing planning (concurrent planning).[1]

Just-in-Time Logistics (or Quick Response)

The process of minimizing the times required to source, handle, produce, transport, and deliver products to meet customer requirements.[1]

Kaizen

A Japanese term for improvement. Continuing improvement involving everyone including managers and workers. In manufacturing, *kaizen* relates to finding and eliminating waste in machinery, labor, or production methods.[1]

Kanban

Japanese word for visible record, loosely translated means card, billboard, or sign. Popularized by Toyota Corporation, it uses standard containers or lot sizes to deliver needed parts to the assembly line just in time for use. [1]

Key Performance Indicator (KPI)

A measure of strategic importance to a company or department. For example, a supply chain flexibility metric is supplier on-time delivery performance, which indicates the percentage of orders fulfilled on or before the original requested date. *See Scorecard.*[1]

Kitting

Light assembly of components or parts into defined units, reducing the need to maintain an inventory of prebuilt, completed products, but increasing the time and labor consumed at shipment.[1]

Landed Cost (also called Total Landed Cost of Net Landed Costs)

Cost of product plus relevant logistics costs such as transportation, warehousing, handling, etc.[1]

Lead Time

The total time that elapses between an order's placement and its receipt. It includes the time required for order transmittal, order processing, order preparation, and transit.[1]

Life Cycle Cost

In cost accounting, a product's life cycle is the period starting with the initial product conceptualization and ending with the withdrawal of the product from the marketplace and final disposition. A product life cycle is characterized by certain defined stages including research, development, introduction, maturity, decline, and abandonment. Life cycle cost is the accumulated costs incurred by a product during these stages.[1]

Logistics

The process of planning, implementing, and controlling procedures for the efficient and effective storage of goods, services, and related information from the point of origin to the point of consumption for the purpose of conforming to customer requirements including inbound, outbound, internal, and external movements.[1]

Logistics Management

Logistics management is that part of supply chain management that plans, implements, and controls the efficient, effective forward-and-reverse flow and storage of goods, services, and related information between the point of origin and the point of consumption to meet customers' requirements. Logistics management activities typically include inbound and outbound transportation management, fleet management, warehousing, materials handling, order fulfillment, logistics network design, inventory management, supply/demand planning, and management of third party logistics services providers. To varying degrees, the logistics function also includes sourcing and procurement, production planning and scheduling, packaging and assembly, and customer service. It is involved in all levels of planning and execution—strategic, operational, and tactical. Logistics management is an integrating function that coordinates and optimizes all logistics activities with other functions including marketing, sales, manufacturing, finance, and information technology.[10]

Low-Unit-of-Measure (LUM) Distribution

In contrast to the traditional bulk model of shipping inventory in full-case quantities to hospital storerooms and subsequently to patient care areas, low-unit-of-measure (LUM) or best-unit-of-measure (BUM) distribution involves breaking cases into smaller units, which are delivered directly to patient areas.[11]

Management Services Organization (MSO)

An entity, either freestanding or sponsored by a hospital or health system, that provides managerial, administrative, and support services (which may include real estate) to medical practices, or to the hospital and its affiliated physicians in conjunction with a capitation contract with a health maintenance organization.[2]

Manufacturing Lead Time

The total time required to manufacture an item, exclusive of lower-level purchasing lead time. For make-to-order products, it is the length of time between the release of an order to the production process and shipment to the final customer. For make-to-stock products, it is the length of time between the release of an order to the production process and receipt into finished goods inventory. Included are order preparation time, queue time, setup time, run time, move time, inspection time, and put-away time. **Synonym: Manufacturing Cycle Time.**[1]

Market Demand

In marketing, the total demand that would exist within a defined customer group in a given geographical area during a particular time period, given a known marketing program.[1]

Material Acquisition Costs

One of the elements comprising a company's total supply chain management costs. These costs consist of the following:

Materials (Commodity) Management and Planning: all costs associated with the supplier sourcing, contract negotiation and qualification, and the preparation, placement, and tracking of a purchase order, including all costs related to buyer/planners.

Supplier Quality Engineering: the costs associated with the determination, development/certification, and monitoring of suppliers' capabilities to fully satisfy the applicable quality and regulatory requirements.

Inbound Freight and Duties: freight costs associated with the movement of material from a vendor to the buyer, including all associated administrative tasks. Duties are those fees and taxes levied by government for moving purchased material across international borders. Customs broker fees should also be included in this category.

Receiving and Put Away: all costs associated with taking possession of material and storing it. **Note:** Inventory-carrying costs are normally covered in a separate worksheet.

Incoming Inspection: All costs associated with the inspection and testing of received materials to verify compliance with specifications.[1]

Materials Management

Inbound logistics from suppliers through the production process. The movement and management of materials and products from procurement through production.[1]

Materials Management Information System (MMIS)

An information system in which authorized users can obtain and/or update the status of all materials. The focus of any materials management information system is to deliver significant improvements in the ability of hospital facilities, networks, and other healthcare organizations to optimize the processes and work flows associated with product sourcing, bidding, end-user requisitioning, usage reporting, and inventory balancing. Effective use of materials management systems assist in quantifying and reducing costs related to inventory, durable medical equipment, pharmaceuticals, and supply chain management.[2]

Meaningful Use

In the context of health information technology, the US Congress defined meaningful use as 1) the use of certified electronic health record (EHR) technology, 2) a certified EHR that is connected in a manner that provides for the electronic exchange of health information to improve care, and 3) provider submission of information on clinical quality measures to the Centers for Medicare & Medicaid Services (CMS). The HITECH Act of the American Recovery and Reinvestment Act provides for Medicare and Medicaid incentive payments to eligible providers that are "meaningful users" of EHR technology. CMS is charged with further defining the criteria for demonstrating meaningful use of EHRs through rulemaking.[2]

National Committee for Quality Assurance (NCQA)

A not-for-profit organization that reviews the performance of health maintenance organizations and other managed care plans, primarily through its formal accreditation program and a group of managed care performance indicators called HEDIS (Health Plan Employer Data and Information Set). NCQA also establishes standards for and certifies primary care practices operating as Patient-Centered Medical Homes. This recognition program, which originally began in 2008 and has continued with the release of updated standards in 2011, established standards around organizing care, working in teams, coordinating and tracking care over time, and using electronic systems to promote continuity. *See Patient-Centered Medical Homes (PCMH).*[2]

Net Assets

Total net assets are calculated as [Total Assets]−[Total Liabilities]; where the total assets are made up of fixed assets (plant, machinery, and equipment) and current assets, which is the total of stock, debtors, and cash (also includes A/R, inventory, prepaid assets, deferred assets, intangibles, and goodwill). The total liabilities are made up in much the same way as long-term liabilities and current liabilities (includes A/P, accrued expenses, and deferred liabilities).[1]

Obsolete Inventory

Inventory for which there is no forecast demand expected. A condition of being out-of-date. A loss of value occasioned by new developments that place the older property at a competitive disadvantage.[1]

Order Cycle

The time and process involved from the placement of an order to the receipt of the order.[1]

Order Management Costs

One of the elements comprising a company's total supply chain management costs. These costs consist of the following:

New Product Release Phase In and Maintenance: This includes costs associated with releasing new products to the field, maintaining released products, assigning product ID, defining configurations and packaging, publishing availability schedules, release letters and updates, and maintaining product databases.

Create Customer Order: This includes costs associated with creating and pricing configurations to order and preparing customer order documents.

Order Entry and Maintenance: This includes costs associated with maintaining the customer database, credit check, accepting new orders, and adding them to the order system, as well as later order modifications.

Contract/Program and Channel Management: This includes costs related to contract negotiation, monitoring progress, and reporting against the customer's contract, including administration of performance or warranty-related issues.

Installation Planning: This includes costs associated with installation engineering, scheduling and modification, handling cancellations, and planning the installation.

Order Fulfillment: This includes costs associated with order processing, inventory allocation, ordering from internal or external suppliers, shipment scheduling, order status reporting, and shipment initiation.

Distribution: This includes costs associated with warehouse space and management, finished goods receiving and stocking, processing shipments, picking and consolidating, selecting carriers, and staging products/systems.

Transportation, Outbound Freight, and Duties: This includes costs associated with all company-paid freight duties from point of manufacturer to end customer or channel.

Installation: This includes costs associated with verification of site preparation, installation, certification, and authorization of billing.

Customer Invoicing/Accounting: This includes costs associated with invoicing, processing customer payments, and verification of customer receipt.[1]

Order Picking
Assembling a customer's order from items in storage.[1]

Order Processing
Activities associated with filling customer orders.[1]

Ordering Cost
The cost of placing an inventory order with a supplier.[1]

Origin
The place where a shipment begins its movement.[1]

Original Equipment Manufacturer (OEM)

A manufacturer that buys and incorporates another supplier's products into its own products. Also products supplied to the original equipment manufacturer or sold as part of an assembly. For example, an engine may be sold to an OEM for use as that company's power source for its generator units.[1]

Outsource

To utilize a third party provider to perform services previously performed in house. Examples include manufacturing of products and call center/customer support.[1]

Patient-Centered Care

In its landmark 2001 report, *Crossing the Quality Chasm,* the Institute of Medicine (IOM) named patient-centered care as one of the six fundamental aims of the US healthcare system. The IOM defines patient-centered care as: Healthcare that establishes a partnership among practitioners, patients, and their families (when appropriate) to ensure that decisions respect patients' wants, needs, and preferences and that patients have the education and support they need to make decisions and participate in their own care. A high degree of consensus exists regarding the key attributes of patient-centered care. In a systematic review of nine models and frameworks for defining patient-centered care, the following six core elements were identified most frequently: education and shared knowledge; involvement of family and friends; collaboration and team management; sensitivity to nonmedical and spiritual dimensions of care; respect for patient needs and preferences; free flow and accessibility of information.[12]

Patient-Centered Medical Home (PCMH)

A collaborative and comprehensive approach to delivering primary care that involves partnerships between patients, their providers, and all those involved in the care delivery process. The PCMH model of care aims to provide the optimal level of quality primary care that is integrated, coordinated, and patient-centered as well as cost-efficient. The National Committee for Quality Assurance (NCQA) and the Joint Commission have set standards for eligible outpatient primary care practices to apply for and receive recognition as an NCQA PCMH.[2]

Pay for Performance

The practice of an insurer (Medicaid, Medicare, private insurer, or managed care company) providing additional payment or not reducing or withholding payment to healthcare practitioners (physicians, hospitals, nursing homes, or home care agencies) if they meet or exceed performance thresholds for providing quality care to patients. The thresholds or measures are generally based on evidence-based practices and can include outcome, process, or structure measures. *See Value-Based Purchasing (VBP).*[2]

Payer

A government agency, insurer, or health plan that pays for healthcare services.[2]

Performance Measures

Indicators of the work performed and the results achieved in an activity, process, or organizational unit. Performance measures should be both nonfinancial and financial. Performance measures enable periodic comparison and benchmarking. *See Performance Measurement Program.*[1]

Performance Measurement Program

A performance measurement program goes beyond just having performance metrics in place. Typical characteristics of a good performance measurement program include the following: metrics that are aligned to strategy and linked to the shop floor or line-level workers: a process and culture that drives performance and accountability to deliver performance against key performance indicators; an incentive plan that is tied to performance goals, objectives, and metrics; and tools/technology in place to support easy data collection and use.[1]

Periodic Automatic Replacement (PAR)

Also Periodic Automatic Replenishment

The numerical amount of inventory or supply items to be maintained at a specific location or the general term designating the level at which to keep the item balance.[13]

Personal Health Record

A computer-accessible, interoperable resource of pertinent health information about an individual. Individuals manage and determine the rights to the access, use, and control of the information in a personal health record. The information originates from multiple sources and is used by individuals and their authorized clinical and wellness professionals to help track individuals' health across multiple providers and over time.[2]

Physical Supply

The movement and storage of raw materials from supply sources to the manufacturing facility.[1]

Physician Preference Item (PPI)

Any patient-care item or medical device for which a physician, nurse, or other clinician could reasonably be expected to express a product preference compared with similar product(s) available from alternative supplier(s); in contrast with a *commodity* item, where similar products are more likely to be viewed by the physician, nurse, or other clinician as functional equivalents of one another. *See Clinical Preference Item (CPI).*[2]

Process Benchmarking

Benchmarking a process (such as the pick, pack, and ship process) against organizations known to be the best in class in this process. Process benchmarking is usually conducted on firms outside of the organization's industry. *See Benchmarking.*[1]

Procurement

The business functions of procurement: planning, purchasing, inventory control, traffic, receiving, incoming inspection, and salvage operations. **Synonym: Purchasing.**[1]

Proof of Delivery (POD)

Information supplied by the carrier containing the name of the person who signed for the shipment, the time and date of delivery, and other shipment delivery-related information. POD is also sometimes used to refer to the process of printing materials just prior to shipment (print on demand).[1]

Purchase Order (PO)

The purchaser's authorization used to formalize a purchase transaction with a supplier. The physical form or electronic transaction a buyer uses when placing an order for merchandise.[1]

Purchasing

The functions associated with buying goods and services a firm requires.[1]

Quality

Conformance to requirements or fitness for use. Quality can be defined through five principal approaches: 1) transcendent quality is an ideal, a condition of excellence, 2) product-based quality is based on a product attribute, 3) user-based quality is fitness for use, 4) manufacturing-based quality is conformance to requirements, and 5) value-based quality is the degree of excellence to an acceptable price. Also, quality has two major components: quality of conformance, where quality is defined by the absence of defects, and quality of design, where quality is measured by the degree of customer satisfaction with a product's characteristics and features.[1]

Quality Control

The management function that attempts to ensure that goods or services a firm manufactures or purchases meet the product or service specifications.[1]

Quality Improvement (QI)

In the context of healthcare, a process or set of activities to maintain and improve the level of care provided to patients. These activities may include reviews, formal measurements, and corrective actions. QI is a standard part of institutional healthcare providers' and health insurance plans' activities. Certain programmatic QI requirements are mandated by law and regulation.[2]

Radio Frequency (RF)

A form of wireless communications that lets users relay information via electromagnetic energy waves from a terminal to a base station that is linked, in turn, to a host computer. The terminal can be placed at a fixed station, mounted on a forklift truck, or carried in a worker's hand. The base station contains a transmitter and receiver for communication with the terminal. RF systems use either narrow-band or spread-spectrum transmissions. Narrow-band data transmissions move along a single limited radio frequency while spread-spectrum transmissions move across several different frequencies. When combined with a bar code system of identifying inventory items, a radio frequency system can relay data instantly, thus updating inventory records in so-called real time.[1]

Radio Frequency Identification (RFID)

The use of radio frequency technology such as RFID tags and tag readers to identify objects. Objects may include virtually anything physical such as equipment, pallets of stock, or even individual units of product.[1]

Receiving Dock

Distribution center location where the actual physical receipt of the purchased material from the carrier occurs.[1]

Reengineering

A fundamental rethinking and radical redesign of business processes to achieve dramatic improvements in performance; a term used to describe the process of making (usually) significant and major revisions or modifications to business processes; also called Business Process Reengineering.[1]

Regional Health Information Organization (RHIO)

A multistakeholder governance entity that convenes nonaffiliated health and healthcare-related providers and the beneficiaries they serve to improve healthcare for the communities in which it operates. RHIOs take responsibility for the processes that enable the electronic exchange of interoperable health information within a defined contiguous geographic area.[2]

Relative Value Units (RVUs)

Units used in the Medicare program's physician fee schedule to reflect the relative resources required to furnish various services. Three component RVUs reflecting work, practice expense, and malpractice expense are combined to form a single RVU for each physician service. The Balanced Budget Act of 1997 provided for a four-year transition period, beginning in January 1999, to convert the practice expense RVU from one based on historical charges to a more resource-based methodology that would reflect actual costs incurred in delivering various services. *See Resource-Based Relative Value Scale (RBRVS).*[2]

Replenishment

The process of moving or resupplying inventory from a reserve (or upstream) storage location or facility to a primary (or downstream) storage or picking location, or to another mode of storage in which picking is performed.[1]

Request for Information (RFI)

A document used to solicit information about vendors, products, and services prior to a formal RFQ/RFP process.[1]

Request for Proposal (RFP)

A document that provides information concerning a manufacturer's needs and requirements. This document is created to solicit proposals from potential suppliers. For example, a computer manufacturer may use an RFP to solicit proposals from suppliers of third-party logistics services.[1]

Request for Quote (RFQ)

A document used to solicit vendor responses when a product has been selected and price quotations are needed from several vendors.[1]

Resource-Based Relative Value Scale (RBRVS)

The classification system that is the basis for the Medicare physician fee schedule. The system assigns to physician services relative value units that incorporate resource consumption for 1) a work component that reflects the physician's skill and time required in furnishing the service, 2) a practice expense component that reflects general practice expenses, such as office rent and wages of personnel, and 3) a malpractice expense component. *See Relative Value Units (RVUs)*.[2]

Returns Inventory Costs

Costs associated with managing inventory returned for any of the following reasons: repair, refurbishment, excess, obsolescence, end of life, ecological conformance, and demonstration. Includes all applicable elements of the Level 2 component inventory carrying cost of total supply chain management cost.[1]

Returns Material Acquisition, Finance, Planning, and IT Costs

The costs associated with acquiring the defective products and materials for repairing or refurbishing items, plus any finance, planning, and information technology costs to support return activity. Includes all applicable elements of the Level 2 components material acquisition cost (acquiring materials for repairs), supply chain–related finance and planning costs, and supply chain management cost.[1]

Revenue Cycle

In the context of hospital reimbursement, the life cycle of payment for a hospital bill, including the various provider functions that must succeed to ensure proper and timely payment for services rendered. The revenue cycle typically begins with provider personnel activities that ensure all required authorizations and referrals have been secured, verify a patient's eligibility for health insurance and benefits, and notify a plan of a patient's admission or the commencement of services. The revenue cycle also includes the activities of utilization management/case management personnel responsible for providing clinical reviews of the patient's care to plan representatives, appealing any denials of coverage resulting from the plan's determination that care was not medically necessary, and following up on such appeals. Billing and receivables staff are further responsible for billing, collecting, and following up on accounts to ensure proper payment. Provider staff responsible for negotiating contracts with private payers also play a key role in the revenue cycle by ensuring that contractual terms protect the provider to the extent possible from inappropriate payment denials.[2]

Risk

In the context of healthcare finance, the chance that the cost of services will differ from the prospective payments made for those services. For example, a health plan incurs a risk in accepting a premium to provide healthcare services to an enrollee of the plan. Similarly, a provider incurs a risk in accepting capitation from a health plan to provide those services.[2]

Root Cause Analysis

A quality improvement process and tool with broad application used for identifying the basic or causal factors underlying variation in performance, including the occurrence or possible occurrence of adverse events. Root cause analysis focuses primarily on systems and processes, not individual performance, and is designed to identify ways to prevent the recurrence of an adverse event. The Joint Commission requires hospitals to conduct root cause analyses for specified sentinel events. *See Joint Commission, The (TJC).*[2]

Safe Harbors

Regulations created by the Office of the Inspector General that immunize from criminal and civil prosecution certain payment and business practices that might otherwise be considered violations of the federal Anti-Kickback Law, as long as various conditions are satisfied. To be protected by a safe harbor, an arrangement must fit squarely in the safe harbor, but failure to comply with a safe harbor provision does not mean that an arrangement is necessarily illegal. Compliance with safe harbors is voluntary, and arrangements that do not comply with a safe harbor must be analyzed on a case-by-case basis for compliance with the Anti-Kickback statute. The safe harbors address, among other things, space and equipment rental arrangements, personal service and management contracts, and payments made by vendors to group purchasing organizations. *See Anti-Kickback Law; Group Purchasing Organization.*[2]

Scorecard

A performance measurement tool used to capture a summary of the key performance indicators (KPIs)/metrics of a company. Metrics dashboards/scorecards should be easy to read and usually have red, yellow, green indicators to flag when the company is not meeting its metrics targets. Ideally, a dashboard/scorecard should be crossfunctional in nature and include both financial and nonfinancial measures. In addition, scorecards should be reviewed regularly—at least on a monthly basis and weekly in key functions, such as manufacturing and distribution, where activities are critical to the success of a company. The dashboard/scorecards philosophy can also be applied to external supply chain partners, such as suppliers, to ensure that their objectives and practices align. **Synonym: Dashboard.**[1]

Security Rule

The provisions of Health Insurance Portability and Accountability Act and related regulations that establish the standards, requirements, and implementation specifics of administrative, physical, and technical safeguards with which covered entities and business associates must comply to ensure the security of electronic protected health information.[2]

Serial Number

A unique number assigned for identification to a single piece that will never be repeated for similar pieces. Serial numbers are usually applied by the manufacturer but can be applied at other points by the distributor or wholesaler. Serial numbers can be used to support traceability and warranty programs.[1]

Shared Services

Consolidation of a company's back-office processes to form a spinout (or a separate "shared services" unit to be run like a separate business), providing services to the parent company and sometimes to external customers. Shared services typically lower overall cost due to the consolidation and may improve support as a result of focus.[1]

Shipping

The function that performs the tasks for the outgoing shipment of parts, components, and products. It includes packaging, marking, weighing, and loading for shipment.[1]

Shrinkage

Reductions of actual quantities of items in stock, in process, or in transit. The loss may be caused by scrap, theft, deterioration, evaporation, etc.[1]

Single-Payer System

A term used to describe a healthcare system under which healthcare insurance for an entire population is provided through a single insurer. Under such a system, healthcare providers submit claims for all patient services to a single payer, which is generally a government agency or a government-contracted third-party administrator.[2]

Six-Sigma Quality

A term generally used to indicate that a process is well controlled (i.e., tolerance limits are 6σ sigma [3.4 defects per million events] from the centerline in a control chart). The term is usually associated with Motorola, which named one of its key operations initiatives Six-Sigma Quality.[1]

Stark Law

A federal law, named for its sponsor, US Congressman Pete Stark (D-CA), which prohibits physician self-referral for Medicare and Medicaid services. Specifically, the law prohibits a physician from referring a patient to a medical facility in which he or she has a financial interest. The Stark Law is implemented through an elaborate series of federal regulations, which include a series of exceptions under which physicians can maintain legitimate business relationships with entities with which they have a financial relationship.[2]

Statement of Work (SOW)

A description of products to be supplied under a contract. A good practice is for companies to have SOWs in place with their trading partners, especially for all top suppliers. In project management, the first project-planning document that should be prepared. It describes the purpose, history, deliverables, and measurable success indicators for a project. It captures the support required from the customer and identifies contingency plans for events that could throw the project off course. Because the project must be sold to management, staff, and review groups, the statement of work should be a persuasive document.[1]

Stock-Keeping Unit (SKU)

A category of unit with a unique combination of form, fit, and function (i.e., unique components held in stock).

> *To illustrate:* If two items are indistinguishable to the customer, or if any distinguishing characteristics visible to the customer are not important to the customer so that the customer believes the two items to be the same, these two items are part of the same SKU.

> *As a further illustration:* Consider a computer company that allows customers to configure a complete computer from a selection of

standard components. For example, they can choose from three keyboards, three monitors, and three CPUs. Customers may also individually buy keyboards, monitors, and CPUs. If the stock were held at the configuration component level, the company would have 9 SKUs. If the company stocks at the component level, the company would have 36 SKUs ([9 component SKUs]+[3*3*3 configured product SKUs]). If, as part of a promotional campaign, the company also specially packaged the products, the company would have a total of 72 SKUs.[1]

Subacute Care
A level of care usually requiring a length of stay longer than short-term acute care and shorter than long-term skilled nursing care. An organized program of care for patients with either intense rehabilitative or medically complex needs, subacute care focuses on achieving specified measurable outcomes using an interdisciplinary case-management approach and providing care in an efficient and low-cost manner.[2]

Subcontracting
Sending production work outside to another manufacturer. This can involve specialized operations such as plating metals or complete functional operations. *See Outsource.*[1]

Sunk Cost
The unrecovered balance of an investment. It's a cost already paid that is not relevant to a decision being made concerning the future. Capital already invested that for some reason cannot be retrieved. A past cost that has no relevance with respect to future receipts and disbursements of a facility undergoing an economic study. This concept implies that since a past outlay is the same regardless of the alternative selected, it should not influence the choice between alternatives.[1]

Supplier

A provider of goods or services. A seller with whom the buyer does business, as opposed to vendor, which is a generic term referring to all sellers in the marketplace. *See Vendor.*[1]

Supplier Certification

Certification procedures verifying that a supplier operates, maintains, improves, and documents effective procedures relating to the customer's requirements. Such requirements can include cost, quality, delivery, flexibility, maintenance, safety, and ISO quality and environmental standards.[1]

Supplier-Owned Inventory

A variant of vendor-managed inventory and consignment inventory. In this case, the supplier not only manages the inventory but also owns the stock close to or at the customer location until the point of consumption or usage by the customer.[1]

Supply Chain

Starting with unprocessed raw materials and ending with the final customer using the finished goods, the supply chain links many companies together; the material and informational interchanges in the logistical process, stretching from acquisition of raw materials to delivery of finished products to the end user. All vendors, service providers, and customers are links in the supply chain.[1]

Supply Chain Design

The determination of how to structure a supply chain. Design decisions include the selection of partners, the location and capacity of warehouse and production facilities, the products, the modes of transportation, and supporting information systems.[1]

Supply Chain Execution (SCE)

The ability to move the product out of the warehouse door. This is a critical capacity and one that only brick-and-mortar firms bring to the B2B table.

Dot-coms have the technology, but that's only part of the equation. The need for SCE drives the dot-coms to offer equity partnerships to wholesale distributors.[1]

Supply Chain Event Management (SCEM)

SCEM is an application that supports control processes for managing events within and between companies. It consists of integrated software functionality that supports five business processes: monitor, notify, simulate, control, and measure supply chain activities.[1]

Supply Chain Integration (SCI)

Likely to become a key competitive advantage of selected e-marketplaces. Similar concept to the back-end integration, but with greater emphasis on the moving of goods and services.[1]

Supply Chain Inventory Visibility

Software applications that permit monitoring events across a supply chain. These systems track and trace inventory globally on a line-item level and notify the user of significant deviations from the plans. Companies are provided with realistic estimates of when the material will arrive.[1]

Supply Chain Management (SCM)

Supply chain management encompasses the planning and management of all activities involved in sourcing and procurement, conversion, and all logistics management activities. Importantly, it also includes coordination and collaboration with channel partners, which can be suppliers, intermediaries, third-party service providers, and customers. In essence, supply chain management integrates supply and demand management within and across companies. Supply chain management is an integrating function primarily responsible for linking major business functions and business processes within and across companies into a cohesive, high-performing business model. It includes all of the logistics management activities noted above, as well as manufacturing operations, and it drives coordination of processes and activities with and across marketing, sales, product design, finance, and information technology.[6]

Supply Chain Network Design Systems

The systems employed in optimizing the relationships among the various elements of the supply chain manufacturing plants, distribution centers, points of sale, as well as raw materials, relationships among product families, and other factors to synchronize supply chains at a strategic level.[1]

Supply Chain–Related Finance and Planning Cost Element

One of the elements comprising a company's total supply chain management costs. These costs consist of supply chain finance costs—costs associated with paying invoices, auditing physical counts, performing inventory accounting, and collecting accounts receivable. Does not include customer invoicing/accounting costs.[1]

Supply Chain–Related IT Costs

Information technology (IT) costs (in US dollars) associated with major supply chain management processes as described below. These costs should include: *development costs* (costs incurred in process reengineering, planning, software development, installation, implementation, and training associated with new and/or upgraded architecture, infrastructure, and systems to support the described supply chain management processes); *execution costs* (operating costs to support supply chain process users, including computer and network operations, EDI and telecommunications services, and amortization/depreciation of hardware); and *maintenance costs* (costs incurred in problem resolution, troubleshooting, repair, and routine maintenance associated with installed hardware and software for described supply chain management processes. Includes costs associated with database administration systems configuration control, release planning, and management). These costs are associated with the following processes:

Plan: **Product Data Management**—product phase in/phase out and release, post-introduction support and expansion, testing and evaluation, and end-of-life inventory management. Item master definition and control.

Forecasting and Demand/Supply Manage and Finished Goods— forecasting, end-item inventory planning, DRP, production master scheduling for all products, and all channels.

Source: **Sourcing/Material Acquisition** — material requisitions, purchasing, supplier quality engineering, inbound freight management, receiving, incoming inspection, component engineering, tooling acquisition, and accounts payable.

Component and Supplier Management—part number cross-references, supplier catalogs, and approved vendor lists.

Inventory Management—perpetual and physical inventory controls and tools.

Make: **Manufacturing Planning**—MRP, production scheduling, tracking, manufacturing engineering, manufacturing documentation management, and inventory/obsolescence tracking.

Inventory Management—perpetual and physical inventory controls and tools. *Manufacturing Execution*—MES detailed and finite interval scheduling, process controls, and machine scheduling.

Deliver: **Order Management**—order entry/maintenance, quotes, customer database, product/price database, accounts receivable, credits and collections, and invoicing.

Distribution and Transportation Management—DRP, shipping, freight management, and traffic management.

Inventory Management—perpetual and physical inventory controls and tools. *Warehouse Management*—finished goods, receiving and stocking, and pick/pack.

Channel Management—promotions, pricing and discounting, and customer satisfaction surveys.

Field Service/Support—field service, customer and field support, technical service, service/call management, returns, and warranty tracking.

***External Electronic Interface:* Plan/Source/Make/Deliver**—interfaces, gateways, and data repositories created and maintained to exchange supply chain–related information with the outside world. E-commerce initiatives. Includes development and implementation costs.

> *Note:* Accurate assignment of IT-related cost is challenging. It can be done using activity-based costing methods or using other approaches such as allocation based on user counts, transactions counts, or departmental head counts. The emphasis should be on capturing all costs. Costs for any outsourced IT activities should be included.[1]

Supply Chain Strategic Planning

The process of analyzing, evaluating, and defining supply chain strategies including network design, manufacturing and transportation strategy, and inventory policy.[1]

Supply Planning

The process of identifying, prioritizing, and aggregating, as a whole with constituent parts, all sources of supply that are required and add value in the supply chain of a product or service at the appropriate level, horizon, and interval. [1]

Supply Warehouse

A warehouse that stores raw materials. Goods from different suppliers are picked, sorted, staged, or sequenced at the warehouse to assemble plant orders.[1]

SWOT Analysis

An analysis of the strengths, weaknesses, opportunities, and threats of and to an organization. SWOT analysis is useful in developing strategy.[1]

Terms and Conditions (Ts & Cs)

All the provisions and agreements of a contract.[1]

Total Cost of Ownership (TCO)

Total cost of a computer asset throughout its life cycle from acquisition to disposal. TCO is the combined hard and soft costs of owning networked information assets. "Hard" costs include items such as the purchase price of the asset, implementation fees, upgrades, maintenance, contracts, support contracts, disposal costs, and license fees that may or may not be up-front or charged annually. These costs are considered "hard" because they are tangible and easily accounted for.[1]

Total Supply Chain Management Cost (five elements)

Total cost to manage order processing, acquire materials, manage inventory, and manage supply chain finance, planning, and IT costs as represented as a percentage of revenue. Accurate assignment of IT-related cost is challenging. It can be done using activity-based costing methods or more traditional approaches. Allocation based on user counts, transaction counts, or departmental headcounts are reasonable approaches. The emphasis should be on capturing all costs, whether incurred in the entity completing the survey or in a supporting organization on behalf of the entity. Reasonable estimates founded in data were accepted as means to assess overall performance. All estimates reflect fully burdened actuals inclusive of salary, benefits, space and facilities, and general and administrative allocations. **Calculation:** [Order Management Costs + Material Acquisition Costs + Inventory Carrying Costs + Supply Chain–Related Finance and Planning Costs + Total Supply Chain–Related IT Costs]/[Total Product Revenue].[1]

Transactions and Code Sets

Under the Health Insurance Portability and Accountability Act of 1996 (HIPAA), the exchange of specific types of information between two parties to carry out financial or administrative activities related to healthcare. The transactions and code sets are 1) healthcare claims or equivalent counter information, 2) healthcare payment and remittance advice, 3) coordination of benefits, 4) healthcare claim status, 5) enrollment and disenrollment in a health plan, 6) eligibility for a health plan, 7) health plan premium payments, 8) referral certification and authorization, 9) first report or injury, 10) health claims attachments, and 11) other transactions that the US Department of Health and Human Services secretary may prescribe by regulation.[2]

Transparency

The ability to gain access to information without regard to the system's landscape or architecture. An example would be where an online customer could access a vendor's website to place an order and receive availability information supplied by a third-party outsource manufacturer or shipment information from a third-party logistics provider.[1]

Trend

General upward or downward movement of a variable over time, such as demand for a product. Trends are used in forecasting to help anticipate changes in consumption over time.[1]

Trend Forecasting Models

Methods for forecasting sales data when a definite upward or downward pattern exists. Models include double exponential smoothing, regression, and triple smoothing.[1]

Turnover

Typically refers to inventory turnover. In the United Kingdom and certain other countries, turnover refers to annual sales volume. *See Inventory Turns.*[1]

Uncompensated Care

Healthcare services rendered for which providers are not reimbursed, usually because the patients treated are poor and uninsured.[2]

US Department of Health and Human Services (HHS)

The federal agency that oversees many aspects of the nation's healthcare system. HHS includes 11 operating divisions such as the Centers for Medicare & Medicaid Services, the Centers for Disease Control and Prevention, the Health Resources and Services Administration, the US Food and Drug Administration, and the National Institutes of Health. The secretary of HHS is a member of the president's cabinet.[2]

Utilization Review (UR)

A formal review of the delivery of health services to determine medical necessity. UR can be conducted prior to, concurrent with, or subsequent to the delivery of services. Managed care plans use UR to control the type and amount of services that their enrollees receive and may contract with independent UR agents to perform such activities.[2]

Value Analysis

A systematic, objective, evidence-based process for evaluating and reducing supply and procedure expenses by considering alternate products and practices which meet, but do not necessarily exceed, the need while maintaining or improving quality, which is measured by objective quality outcome criteria. Value analysis is customer focused, process-oriented, and driven by outcomes and data.[2]

Value-Based Purchasing (VBP)

A reimbursement methodology under which a portion of a payment rate paid to a provider (e.g., hospital, nursing home, physician) is contingent upon the provider's performance on certain quality measures. Under the Affordable Care Act, Medicare must implement a VBP program beginning in fiscal year 2013, whereby a portion of the acute inpatient hospital payments will be withheld and hospitals can "earn back" an incentive payment based on their performance on prescribed quality metrics, including both process and outcome measures, as well as patient experience of care as identified in the Hospital-Consumer Assessment of Health Plans Survey. High performers will be rewarded with payments that are higher than their withholding, while low performers will experience payment penalties such that payments overall under the program are budget-neutral. The amount of the withhold starts at 1% in fiscal year 2013 and will phase in to a maximum of 2% in fiscal year 2017. *See Pay for Performance.*[2]

Value Chain

A series of activities, which, when combined, define a business process; the series of activities from manufacturers to the retail stores that define the industry supply chain.[1]

Value Chain Analysis

A method of identifying all the elements in the linkage of activities a firm relies on to secure necessary materials and services starting from their point of origin to manufacturing and to distribution of their products and services to an end user.[1]

Vendor

The manufacturer or distributor of an item or product line.[1]

Vendor Code

A unique identifier, usually a number and sometimes the company's DUNS number, assigned by a customer for the vendor from which it buys.

> *Example:* A grocery store chain buys Oreo cookies from Nabisco. For accounting purposes, the grocery store chain identifies Nabisco as vendor #76091. One company can have multiple vendor codes.

> *Example:* Welch's Foods sells many different products—frozen grape juice concentrate, chilled grape juice, bottled grape juice, and grape jelly. Because each of these items is a different type of product (frozen food, chilled food, beverages, dry food), they may also have a different buyer at the grocery store chain, requiring a different vendor code for each product line.[1]

Vendor-Managed Inventory (VMI)

The practice of retailers making suppliers responsible for determining order size and timing, usually based on receipt of retail POS and inventory data. Its goal is to increase retail inventory turns and reduce stock-outs.[1]

Wage Index

The ratio of the average hourly wage rate in a particular labor market, such as a metropolitan statistical area or rural area, to the average hourly wage rate in a larger area, such as the entire United States. The Medicare program uses an area wage index based on hospital wage data to adjust payments under its various prospective payment systems.[2]

Waste

In JIT, any activity that does not add value to the good or service in the eyes of the consumer. A byproduct of a process or task with unique characteristics requiring special management control. Waste production can usually be planned and controlled. Scrap is typically not planned and may result from the same production run as waste.[1]

Endnotes

1. "Glossary of Supply Chain Terms," Inbound Logistics, accessed June 27, 2014, http://www.inboundlogistics.com/cms/logistics-glossary/.

2. Greater New York Hospital Association, *Healthcare Terms 2014–15* (New York: GNYHA: May 2014).

3. "Basing Point Pricing System," Investopedia, accessed March 31, 2015, http://www.investopedia.com/terms/b/basing-point-pricing-system.asp.

4. "Quality Improvement," U.S. Department of Health and Human Services, Health Resources and Services Administration, accessed July 1, 2014. http://www.hrsa.gov/quality/toolbox/methodology/qualityimprovement/.

5. "Cost, Quality, Outcomes Movement," The Association for Healthcare Resource & Materials Management (AHRMM), accessed June 27, 2014, http://www.ahrmm.org/ahrmm/resources_and_tools/cost_quality_outcomes/what_is_cqo.jsp.

6. "Appendix: Common Terms in Health Information Technology," in *Evidence on the Costs and Benefits of Health Information Technology* (Washington, DC: Congress of the United States, Congressional Budget Office: May 2008), http://www.cbo.gov/sites/default/files/05-20-healthit.pdf.

7. "About GS1," GS1 website, accessed July 1, 2014. http://www.gs1.org/about/.

8. "GS1 Healthcare US: Charter Version 3.0," GS1 Healthcare US, accessed June 27, 2014, http://www.gs1us.org/DesktopModules/Bring2mind/DMX/Download.aspx?Command=Core_Download&EntryId=349&PortalId=0&TabId=785.

9. "Global Location Numbers (GLN)," GS1 website, accessed November 17, 2014, http://www.gs1.org/docs/idkeys/GS1_Global_Location_Numbers.pdf.

10. "Glossary of Terms," Council of Supply Chain Management Professionals, accessed March 30, 2015, https://cscmp.org/research/glossary-terms.

11. M. Darling and S. Wise, "Not Your Father's Supply Chain," *Materials Management in Health Care* 19, no. 4 (2010): 4.

12. D. Shaller, *Patient-Centered Care: What Does It Take?* The Commonwealth Fund pub. no. 1067, October 2007, http://www.commonwealthfund.org/usr_doc/Shaller_patient-centeredcarewhat-doesittake_1067.pdf?section=4039.

13. "Lexicon," The Association for Healthcare Resource & Materials Management (AHRMM), accessed December 16, 2014, www.ahrmm.org/lexicon.

Index of Basic Terms